Table of Conte

MW01101487

❖ Acknowledgements iii

❖ Foreword.. v

❖ Introduction: Teena Gudjonson...Biography vii

❖ Simple tips to increase your metabolism and start burning fat today! 1

❖ Getting lean without counting calories 3

❖ What you should know about good fats and carbohydrates...
don't be a phobic!! 7

❖ Your cupboards.... cleaning out the junk and stocking up with the good stuff....13

❖ Fueling for Exercise 15

❖ RECIPE SECTION... 17

    Breakfast Options.. 19

    Lunch and Dinner Options.. 35

    Smoothies.. 91

    Tasty Treats.. 107

VISIT MY WEBSITE FOR GREAT TIPS AND IDEAS!!

teenasfitness.com

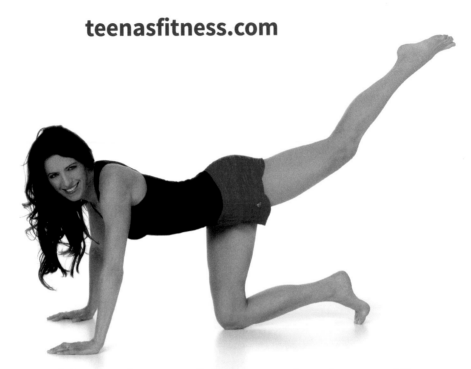

Order an additional copy of this great book as a gift
or buy an E-book version today. Available on Amazon.com,
participating retailers or visit my website.

Order on-line at

www.teenasfitness.com

Visit my Facebook page at **www.facebook.com/www.feellikeafitnessmodel**

ACKNOWLEDGEMENTS

I'd like to thank the many friends, family and clients that inspired me to write this book and put up with all my emails for feedback over the past year! A very special thanks to my husband, brother, sister-in-law and to my children who gave me great encouragement along the way.

Several interior images taken by Jayson Hencheroff of Focal Point Studios, Prince George, B.C.

Remember... Think good, eat good, feel good

FOREWORD

I was motivated to write this book after being asked by dozens of clients to share my recipes and secrets for healthy weight loss. You don't need a pill, a needle, liposuction or great genetics to get the body you've always wanted… all you need to do is re-train your mind and body to eat healthy and stay active. Consistently fueling your body with clean healthy food is sure to give you long-lasting results.

Think eating healthy is boring? Thing again! When I started doing fitness competitions… the only items on my eating plan were poached chicken, fish, plain oats, egg whites, yams and rice. I loved competing but I loved food even more. I knew there had to be a way to incorporate the basics of a fitness diet with the great tasting foods I love… and that's when I started coming up with lean and clean recipes. My recipes not only suited my personal endeavors but also became a way of eating for my whole family.

All of the information indicated in this Fitness Recipe Book is based on a combination of my education, trial & error and years of experience as a fitness competitor & personal trainer. I wanted to share my knowledge and offer a book that would give readers all the information and tools necessary to start their journey to permanent weight loss and a healthy lifestyle.

Please remember that information provided is based strongly on my opinions and beliefs… these can vary greatly among fitness professionals. This book is intended for those in good health and should not in any way be mistaken for or replace medical advice. As with any diet or exercise program, individuals should speak with their physician or health care professional prior to engaging in or following the information I've offered in this book.

Based on my own personal experience as well as hearing testimony from dozens of clients over the years; most individuals that follow this type of eating plan feel stronger, healthier, more energetic and happier than ever. Above all, you really can achieve great results and a very lean body when eating a clean diet and combining the right ratios of nutrients.

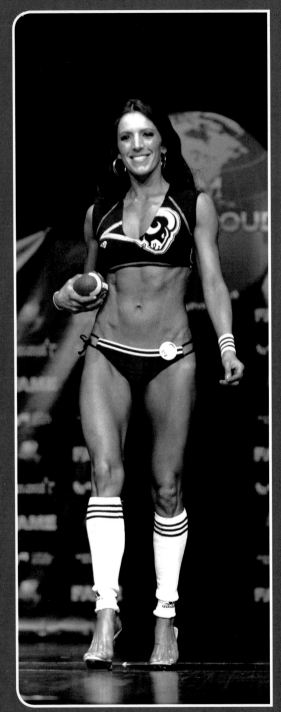
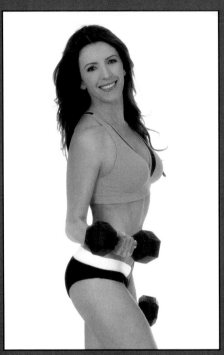
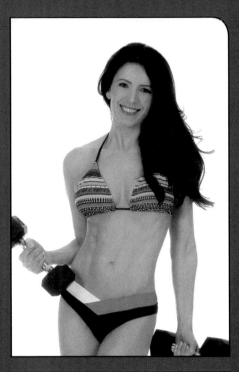
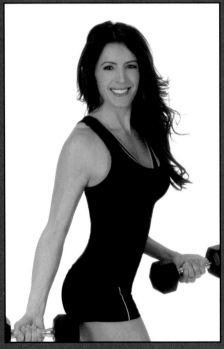
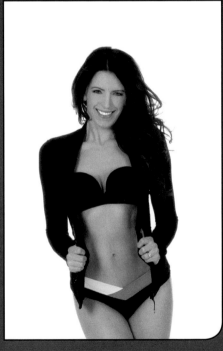

INTRODUCTION

Teena Gudjonson - Biography

Dietary Technologist, Personal Trainer, Fitness Model, Fitness Competitor, Writer, Lifestyle Coach, Wife and Mother. I started off in this industry as a dietary supervisor in a hospital writing diets for patients. Several years later I branched out into Sports Nutrition to expand my knowledge of the human body and how it interacts with the fuel we feed it. I soon took an interest in human kinetics and realized how great of an affect exercise and healthy eating can have on our bodies.

I became fascinated with the ability to manipulate my body through diet and exercise. I'm very passionate about health and fitness as well as helping others. I had always wanted to compete and decided to register for my first competition in 2008 just seven months after giving birth to my second child. I competed in Calgary, Alberta Canada with FAME at a regional show and came in first place in the open fitness model division. From there I obtained my personal trainer certification, opened a gym and have been hooked on fitness ever since.

There's a real science involved in preparing for competition, I love experimenting with the human body…. the possibilities are endless!

MY LIFE LONG GOALS AND PHILOSOPHIES

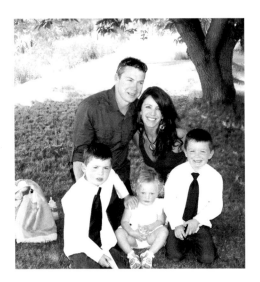

First and foremost my priority is to be an excellent wife and role model for my children. Family is everything… it's my support system and the foundation of my success.

Life long goals include being actively involved in the fitness industry and hopefully making a difference in the lives of others. I've just started my own website and would love to eventually expand my business into marketing healthy food products. I also plan to continue writing articles related to the importance of good nutrition and exercise. Ultimately I'd like to have my very own brand of food products and a series of exercise videos.

I have two philosophies that I try to remind myself of on a daily basis… the first is that ordinary people can do extraordinary things – it's all about hard work, perseverance, and determination. The second is to never take anything for granted and to be thankful each day for everything I have.

I also believe that a healthy lifestyle can be the answer to complete wellness on many different levels. I strongly believe that many of the illnesses in today's society such as problems related to hormonal imbalances, stress, heart disease, type II diabetes, joint & muscle soreness, fatigue and so on can be prevented and improved with proper nutrition and regular exercise. These two powerful tools may in fact be your best defense against chronic disease.

SIMPLE TIPS TO INCREASE YOUR METABOLISM AND START BURNING FAT TODAY!

Over the years I've met many individuals that hadn't previously had any long term success for losing weight or keeping it off. A few of the major issues I found with these individuals was related to their diet. A common myth is that if you cut calories, you will lose weight. This isn't always true. Sometimes people cut calories by too much, skip meals or fill up on non-nutrient dense foods which in fact can make your body go into what us fitness trainers commonly refer to as "starvation mode". For example if you're one of those people that doesn't eat after dinner and skips breakfast but still can't seem to lose weight, it's most likely because your body has slowed down its own metabolic rate. It does this to compensate for the fact that it won't be getting any fuel (food) for the next 15 or 16 hours. Similarly, if you're eating foods that are made up of empty calories that provide very little nutrition, your body is more likely to store these foods as body fat rather than effectively use them as a source of fuel for your body.

A common belief is that weight loss comes down to calories consumed versus calories burned; however, I strongly disagree with this. If one was to consume 1200 empty calories per day in the form of high fat ice cream and cinnamon buns versus 1200 clean calories per day in the form of healthy proteins, carbohydrates and good fats…. not only would your body perform much differently but it's going to look a whole lot different too. The better you fuel your body, the better it will perform and the better it will look. The key to permanent fat loss and a lean physique is to increase your metabolism. Yo-Yo dieting and extreme dietary restrictions will adversely affect your efforts to increase your metabolism permanently.

There are a few simple tricks that I suggest to increase your metabolism, start burning fat and get that lean body you've always wanted;

- ❖ Eat every 2½ to 3 hours throughout the day with your last meal being a small snack including protein approximately 1 hour before bed.

- ❖ Ensure each meal includes lean protein such as chicken or turkey breast meat, lean cuts of beef, egg whites, fish, cottage cheese or whey powder.

- ❖ Ensure each meal includes good carbohydrates such as rice, yams, sweet potatoes, beans, lentils, vegetables or grain such as oatmeal. This is discussed further in the next section.

- ❖ Don't skip meals. Keeping your body fueled throughout the day will keep your blood sugar levels constant and your metabolism boosted.

- ❖ Eat clean. The more wholesome foods you can eat the better. Stay away from processed foods that are pre-cooked, pre-packaged, or canned. Eat fresh, whole foods.

- ❖ Cut sugar out of your diet. Sugar comes in many forms such as syrups, nectars, brown sugar, white sugar, honey, glucose, fructose and so on. Sugars cause a rise in blood sugar levels and are more easily stored as body fat. They are also a very concentrated source of calories that provide very little nutrition regardless of which form they come in. Try using an all-natural sweetener such as Stevia or Truvia instead of sugar.

- ❖ Cut out white flour in the form of white breads, white pancakes, white pasta, enriched wheat flour, donuts, cookies, pastries and all other processed baked goods. Not only do these foods provide very little nutrition for a lot of calories…. they usually come with added toppings such as butter, syrups, jams, and so on.

- ❖ Exercise at least 3 times per week with both cardio and weights. Many people… especially women, tend to think that the more cardio they do the more fat they will lose. Although cardiovascular activity such as running on a treadmill, walking, riding a bike and aerobics will help you to lose weight, lifting weights is generally a much easier way to get a lean and toned body with long-lasting and permanent results. Once you have lean muscle mass (and I don't mean being bulky or stocky), the higher your metabolic rate will be even at times of rest. The higher your metabolism, the more you can eat while still burning body fat and staying lean.

GETTING LEAN WITHOUT COUNTING CALORIES

*A*re you one of those people that are constantly looking at the calorie content of everything you eat? Do you believe that losing weight is merely a matter of calories in versus calories out? If so, you're not alone. Most of my clients have lived their lives counting calories. When they start a diet they tend to have a very definite outlook on how many calories they should be eating in a day. I am convinced that this type of dieting has a negative impact. So how does a person get a really lean body and keep it for life? Let's take a closer look.

Although I don't believe in counting calories, I do believe you should get your calories from clean foods that are rich in complex carbohydrates, lean proteins and healthy fats. This will help to increase your metabolism. The higher your metabolism, the more fat you will burn around the clock… even while resting.

I strongly believe that your body can process clean calories differently than calories from processed and unhealthy foods such as sugary yogurts, pastries, white bread, processed meats and so on. Your body is more likely to store unhealthy calories as body fat rather than using them to maintain lean muscle. Calories from clean foods also offer your body a great source of long lasting energy. Not only are you sure to notice a physical difference in your body but you will also feel great on the inside. Most of my clients who follow these few tips say they "feel better than they've felt in years".

With regards to cutting calories, I would highly recommend that you refrain from cutting your calories too much or starving yourself. Although you can initially get great results, you may quickly re-gain the weight you lost (and then some) as soon as you re-incorporate more calories. I would suggest that you stop counting calories and focus more on the type of calories you are eating rather than the amounts.

As a general rule of thumb, I would never recommend less than 1200 calories for a woman and no less than 2000 for a man (unless a person was unable to perform activity or had a medical consideration). Severely restricting your caloric intake is unsustainable as well as unhealthy and generally leads to a cycle of yo-yo dieting. I also see this in individuals that routinely follow detox programs. Wouldn't it be better if you didn't have to detox because you ate so clean all year round? I like to follow the 80/20 rule… 80% of the time I eat very clean and 20% of the time I allow myself whatever I like.

Over the years I have found that my appetite for unhealthy foods has drastically decreased. The healthier you eat the less your body will crave unhealthy foods. I recall a time when I thought boxed doughnuts and cookies tasted great…not the case anymore.

Another major point in raising your metabolism is how often you eat. I believe that we need to eat every two and a half to three hours (except for when we are at complete rest) to keep our metabolism from slowing down and going into what I call "starvation mode". Starvation mode is a common term used to describe your metabolism slowing down to compensate for lack of calories over several hours. It's not uncommon for some people to go from 7pm to 11am without eating. The body is sure to slow down to compensate for this.

Our bodies and metabolism adjust to the way we fuel it. If you don't consistently fuel your body - how can your body consistently burn calories? Instead, your body will try to hold on to those calories as reserve until the next time you fuel it. I feel permanent weight loss comes from eating five to six smaller meals per day rather than two to three big meals with nothing in between. Your appetite should also decrease naturally if you eat clean foods at regular intervals.

Although eating more often may initially cause you to feel full all the time, your metabolism should quickly adjust to start burning more calories. Within a month or two of eating this way you will most likely start to feel hungrier between meals and may not even be able to last three hours without some food. When I'm really strict with clean eating and regular intervals I find myself waking up hungry in the middle of the night and having to eat something.

Another important topic when it comes to weight loss is sugar. I always use caution with any type of sugar. Not only because I have a strong family history of diabetes but also because I cannot get "competition ready" if I'm consuming too many calories from sugar. This includes natural sugars in the form of brown or cane sugar, honey, fancy molasses, maple syrup, agave nectar or any other sweetener that contains calories.

Many people are under the impression that natural sugars are okay when they are trying to lose weight. While natural ones may be a better choice than white sugar they can still greatly impact your weight loss efforts. Although I use honey, molasses and maple syrup in small amounts (as you will find in some of the recipes), I am careful to consume less calories from sugar when preparing for a fitness competition. Keeping my blood sugar levels constant always provides great results for me.

Alcohol is another big factor in weight loss. Many people will do all the right things when it comes to diet and exercise but continue to drink alcohol on a regular basis. Alcohol contains non-nutrient dense calories that your body doesn't require for bodily functions. These type of calories are easily stored as body fat. I'm not saying that you can never have alcohol if you want to lose weight; however, if you are consuming alcohol 3-4 times a week, you may want to consider cutting back to once or twice per week and trying to find a low calorie beverage. Many people will switch to light beer but then end up drinking twice as many….not a great solution.

So how do you get quick results without counting calories or skipping meals? I find that the most effective and permanent weight loss is achieved by combining a lean protein with every meal. I believe that incorporating good healthy fats and protein with carbohydrates slows the absorption of the carbohydrates rather than quickly storing them as body fat. I also believe that if you are going to have sugars (even the natural sugars from fruit), it is best to have them with a protein or fat source such as cottage cheese or nuts to lower the impact on your blood sugar levels (unless you need the sugar for medical reasons). I have experimented with this for many years… it definitely appears to have a huge impact on how my body responds. I achieve results very quickly when I combine protein with my carbohydrates at meals and can be competition ready in as little as 5-6 weeks. Examples of this would be having oatmeal with egg whites or mixing protein powder into your oatmeal rather than having a bowl of oatmeal with fruit and yogurt. Although some Greek yogurts are high in protein, yogurt generally has more carbohydrates than protein so I tend to use yogurt as my carb at a meal and then combine it with a lean protein such as dry cottage cheese.

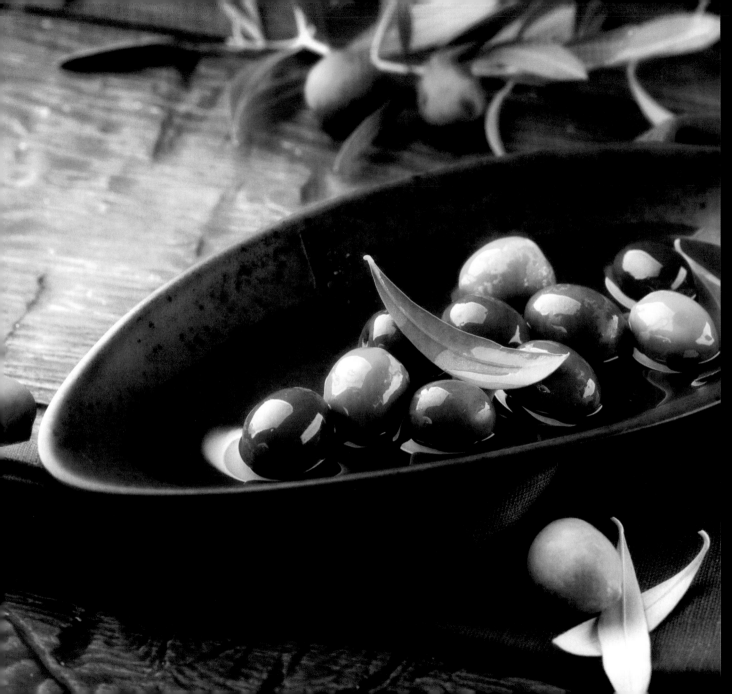

WHAT YOU SHOULD KNOW ABOUT GOOD FATS AND CARBOHYDRATES... DON'T BE A PHOBIC!!

Many people tend to be carb-phobic. The myth that cutting carbs is the best and only way to lose weight quickly and effectively is completely untrue. Although cutting carbs may help you to lose weight in the short term, it is not a reasonable long term solution. Your body needs healthy complex carbohydrates to perform a number of important body functions including regulation of hormones, proper brain function and to provide energy for activity just to name a few.

Cutting carbs for life is nearly impossible, unhealthy and way too boring. I feel it's best to incorporate these nutrient rich foods into each meal and let your body become accustom to using them effectively. Even when fitness competitors are preparing for fitness competitions with their washboard abs and firm bodies... they are consuming many carbohydrates to attain those ripped bodies.

The key is to always combine your carbohydrates with protein and a healthy fat to slow their absorption and to prevent the carbohydrate from being stored as body fat too easily. Also, you want to ensure that you are consuming clean carbohydrates (not processed) in the form of rice, sweet potatoes, yams, oats, quinoa, corn, vegetables, low-sugar yogurt and skim milk.

Although yogurt and milk products contain some protein, they generally provide more carbohydrates by percentage and therefore I count most yogurts and milk as a carbohydrate. For weight loss, you'll want to choose a yogurt with no added sugars and combine it with a protein. The exception to this rule is high protein no-fat Greek yogurt which is generally much higher in protein. Cheese, unless you buy the skim or no fat cheese have a high fat content so when consuming cheese I count it as a fat rather than a protein or carbohydrate. The same is true of almond or peanut butter which people often mistake as a high protein source. Although these contain some protein, they contain much more fat by percentage as well as some carbohydrates.

DON'T BE SCARED OF GOOD FATS

I run into this all the time. Client after client, person after person, that say to me "I can't eat that, it has fat in it". Little do people realize that our bodies require healthy fats to survive and to burn stored body fat. It's not eating fat that makes you fat… it's a combination of everything else including the type of fat you're eating, the amount of sugar you eat, the processed and high calorie/low-nutrient foods you consume and lack of activity that is making you fat. In fact, if you've been buying no-fat or low-fat products in an effort to lose weight and it's not working… it's most likely because you haven't been fueling your body with the healthy fat it needs to increase your metabolism, provide energy for activity and to immobilize your own body fat stores.

As with severely restricting calories and causing your body to go into that "starvation mode" - the same is true if you cut fat from your diet. If you completely cut out fat and don't provide your body with adequate healthy fats… your body will be much more likely to hold onto and store body fat. In addition, healthy fats help to slow the digestion and absorption of other nutrients which helps to keep your blood sugar levels constant which in turn will aid your body to use those calories effectively as a source of energy rather than readily storing them as body fat.

The key is to include clean healthy unsaturated fats into your diet. Providing you don't suffer from heart disease or high cholesterol, you can also consume saturated fats in **small** amounts while still successfully achieving your weight loss goals. Saturated fats are found in foods such as red meat, cheese, coconut oil, butter and egg yolks. Saturated fats are usually solid at room temperature such as butter and generally come from an animal source. Dairy and meat products are sources of saturated fat.

Consumption of saturated fat is the most common dietary cause of increased cholesterol levels; however, weight loss efforts and a lean body can still be achieved while incorporating some saturated fat in your diet, I like to use the 80/20 rule – 80% of the fat I consume is from healthy unsaturated sources and 20% from saturated fat sources. I don't spend time measuring these percentages out. I just use it as a general rule of thumb. For example, having a ½ tsp. of coconut oil or butter on your brown rice or an occasional fatty dinner (prime rib & gravy once per week) isn't going to abolish your weight loss efforts. In fact, once you increase your metabolism you may be able to eat fattier cuts of meat and white pasta more often without gaining weight.

As a general rule of thumb, it is suggested that not more than 15-20% of your calories are coming from fat and that you have plenty of lean protein and complex carbohydrates. For instance, if you were eating fatty hamburger meat nightly rather than lean chicken breasts or white fish… you may be getting more dietary fat than you need without adequate protein. When I'm preparing for fitness competitions, I generally keep my fat calories to 15% of my total caloric intake.

A typical meal for me would be 4oz. chicken breast, ½ cup rice, 6-8 oz. of vegetables and ½ tsp. of olive oil or butter. Again, I don't measure percentages of my fats and so on – I just estimate and make sure that my meal is very healthy with adequate protein and good complex carbs and a little fat – mostly unsaturated. I don't count the little bit of olive oil used to prepare chicken and so on if I'm grilling or pan searing but try not to overdue the oil or deep fry foods (even in good oil).

Good healthy fats include avocado, nuts, all natural peanut or nut butters, olive/flax/grape seed oil, olives, flax seed, healthy fish and so on. See chart on following page for amount of healthy fats found in various foods.

Healthy fats provide you with Omega 3, 6, and 9 essential fatty acids. These are referred to as essential fatty acids and are important for:

▶ Absorption of fat soluble vitamins A,D,E,K.

▶ Maintaining healthy skin, hair and nails.

- ► Good brain function and can help prevent dementia

- ► Cushion and protect our internal organs and can help prevent certain cancers of the organs.

- ► Help us lose weight

    - ❖ Healthy fats are digested slowly which keeps you from feeling hungry and will curb your appetite

    - ❖ Consuming healthy fats will help immobilize your own body fat stores. Your body won't feel the need to hang onto body fat for necessary functions if you're regularly supplying it with good fats.

How to incorporate healthy fats into your diet:

- ► A supplement or capsule. 500 mg/day is considered sufficient but recommendations are always changing so check with your health professional.

- ► Can get Omega 3's from foods we eat such as fatty fish like salmon, lake trout, herring and mackerel as well as things like flax seed and walnuts.

- ► Omegas 6's are found in safflower, sunflower, corn and pumpkin oil. Our consumption of these is generally too high as these oils are found in a variety of products so supplementation is usually not necessary.

- ► Sources of Omega 9's are olives, olive oil, avocados, peanuts, sesame oil and cashews. These are not necessary to incorporate into the diet as your body can manufacture omega 9's if 3's and 6's are present

The following is a chart with a list of healthy fats and the amount of Omega fat they provide – taken from a reliable website.

Food	Omega-3 (grams per100g)	Omega-6 (grams per 100g)
Flax	20.3	4.9
Hemp seeds	7.0	21.0
Pumpkin seeds	3.2	23.4
Salmon	3.2	0.7
Walnuts	3.0	30.6
Grape seed	2.1	9.0
Herring	2.0	0.4
Soybeans	1.2	8.6
Butter	1.2	1.8
Olive oil	0.6	7.9
Wheat germ	0.5	5.5
Sunflower seeds	0	30.7
Almond	0	9.2
Olives	0	1.6

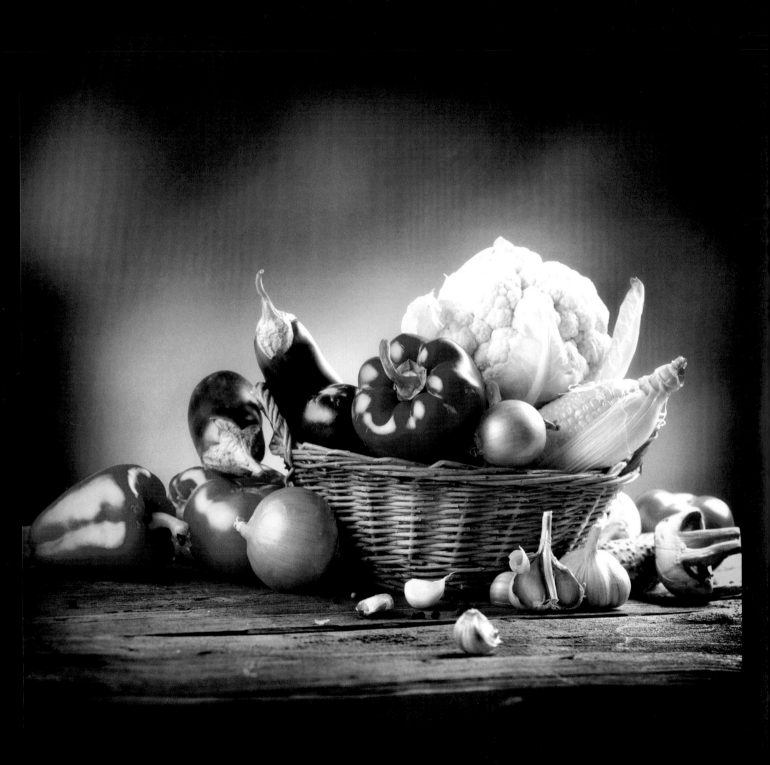

YOUR CUPBOARDS....
CLEANING OUT THE JUNK AND
STOCKING UP WITH THE GOOD STUFF

*T*he secret to long-term success is making sure that you have enough good stuff on hand at all times. Be sure to stock your cupboards with wholesome food items such as the ones mentioned in this section. I recommend having a checklist for the grocery store, making sure you set one day a week aside to shop for groceries and making sure you have everything you need for the week.

I always make sure I have things made up ahead of time. Here are some good ideas for pre-cooking for the week and things to have on hand in the freezer. You can find recipes for these ideas in the recipe section.

❖ Cook a whole pot of rice and a pot of old fashioned oats. Transfer to a glass storage container and keep in the fridge for the week. When you're looking for a quick meal, take out a cup full and heat in the microwave to have for your carbohydrate. Refer to the recipe section - the baked oatmeal squares and quiche are great for this.

❖ I like to cook up a whole chicken or turkey to have fresh meat in the fridge at all times. It's a great way to snack on high protein and in a pinch you can throw your rice, some veggies and turkey or chicken together for a stir-fry at dinner.

❖ Make up a big batch of the protein pancakes and keep some in the fridge and some in the freezer. The ones in the fridge will last all week and if you run out you can grab some from the freezer. This is also great to do with the protein cookies (which can be used as a meal replacement on the run and in place of breakfast if you're in a hurry).

- ❖ I always have some healthy balsamic dressing made up in the fridge or a raspberry yogurt dressing made with Greek yogurt. Put some in a little to-go bottle to take with you when you eat out.

- ❖ When you're making ground chicken breast chili or spaghetti sauce, make extra and freeze in meal size portions. Take out in the morning for those evenings you know you don't have time to cook.

- ❖ Have frozen fruit items for smoothies pre-portioned and frozen in little containers for smoothie recipes such as ½ cup portions of stewed rhubarb, sliced banana, pumpkin puree, berries, etc…

- ❖ Keep items such as egg whites (can buy pure liquid ones), dry or 1% cottage cheese, plain Greek yogurt, skim cheese, and lots of veggies in the fridge at all times.

- ❖ Keep your cupboards stocked with items such as brown rice cakes, all natural peanut butter, canned tuna, chickpeas, lentils, sugar-free pancake syrup, apple sauce, canned pumpkin etc…

- ❖ I like to keep a sugar substitute such as Splenda, Truvia or Stevia on hand. I use the zero calorie ones in baking. Remember that even the healthier types of sugar such as agave nectar and coconut sugar are still high in calories. It's best to avoid processed sugar of all types if you are solely concerned about weight loss but when your sweet tooth gets ahead of you…. try to find low calorie ways to replace sweet treats.

- ❖ Always have low-calorie condiments such as salsa, hot sauce and buffalo sauce on hand.

- ❖ I like to use Unsweetened Almond Milk as an alternative to milk so I keep a case on hand at all times. It is only 40 calories per cup and a great substitute in baking and smoothies.

- ❖ Keep a few all natural ice-pops in the freezer; frozen grapes, frozen raspberries or some frozen sliced bananas for a sweet and refreshing treat when you are craving something cold on a hot day.

FUELING FOR EXERCISE

*A*re you one of those people that exercises a few hours a day several times a week and can't seem to shake those extra pounds? Maybe you've been doing 10km runs five times a week and still can't get the results you're looking for. Many people don't fuel their bodies properly for exercise.

There are a few simple tips I like to follow to maximize my exercise and training efforts;

❖ Unless you are a professional athlete or training for a specific event, 30-40 minutes of cardio 5-6x per week should be adequate for maintaining a lean physique. You will want your cardio sessions to be challenging for you (providing you have no medical condition that prevents you from doing so) and should have variety so that your body never becomes accustom to what it is doing. Whether you are running, biking or hiking outside or doing a cardio machine inside – try to change it up every other day.

❖ Over training with cardio can cause your body to burn your muscle as a source of energy which in turn can lower your metabolism and negatively impact your weight loss efforts.

❖ Don't do your cardio immediately after eating. To maximize fat burning, try doing cardio first thing in the morning before you eat or at least 2 hours after your last meal (unless advised otherwise due to a medical condition).   If you perform cardio immediately after eating, your body will tend to burn the glucose readily available from the food you just ate prior to dipping into your fat stores as a source of energy.

❖ Weight train 3 times per week with weight bearing exercises. This is how you build muscle, increase your metabolism and start burning fat even at rest.

- ❖ Do not do your weight workout on an empty stomach. Your body needs protein, carbohydrates and good fats to build muscle. If you perform weight resistance exercise on an empty stomach, your body will break down your muscle as a source of energy. This is completely counterproductive.

- ❖ Great PRE WORKOUT MEAL would be oatmeal with peanut butter and egg whites on the side or chicken breast with rice & avocado

- ❖ Re-fuel your muscles within an hour of weight resistance training. You want to fill up on protein to refuel those muscles. This is the only meal of the day that I would not include healthy fats as they can slow the uptake of the protein.

- ❖ Great POST WORKOUT MEAL for maximum gains would be a whey protein isolate or concentrate powder shake with skim milk and banana or fruit (See the Smoothie Section). Protein powders are quickly absorbed by the body. You could also have white fish or chicken with yams or rice if you prefer.

For more tips and ideas on exercise visit my website:
teenasfitness.com

The

RECIPE SECTION

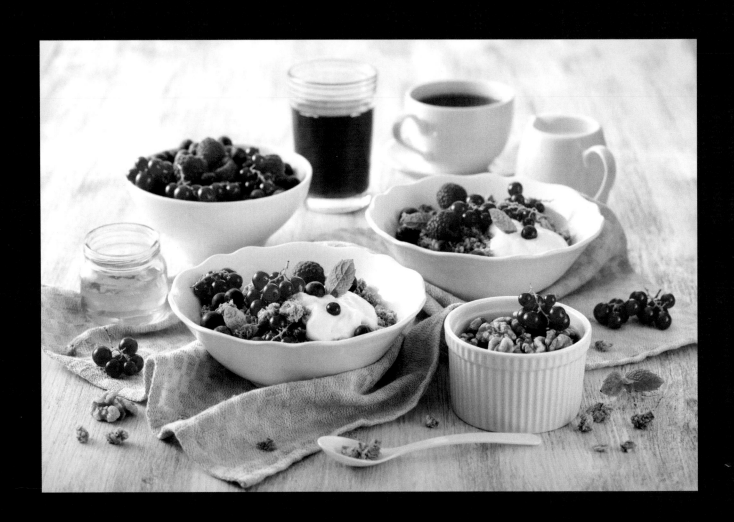

Recipe's for LEAN BREAKFASTS & SNACKS

Options for meals 1 &2 of the day

❖ Baked Oatmeal Squares 21

❖ Healthy Homemade Granola with Greek Yogurt 23

❖ Protein Pancakes 25

❖ Healthy French Toast 27

❖ Spicy Egg Omelete 29

❖ Spicy Spinach Mini Quiche 30

❖ Egg McHealthins 31

❖ Protein Packed Bowls 32

❖ Protein Energy Bars 33

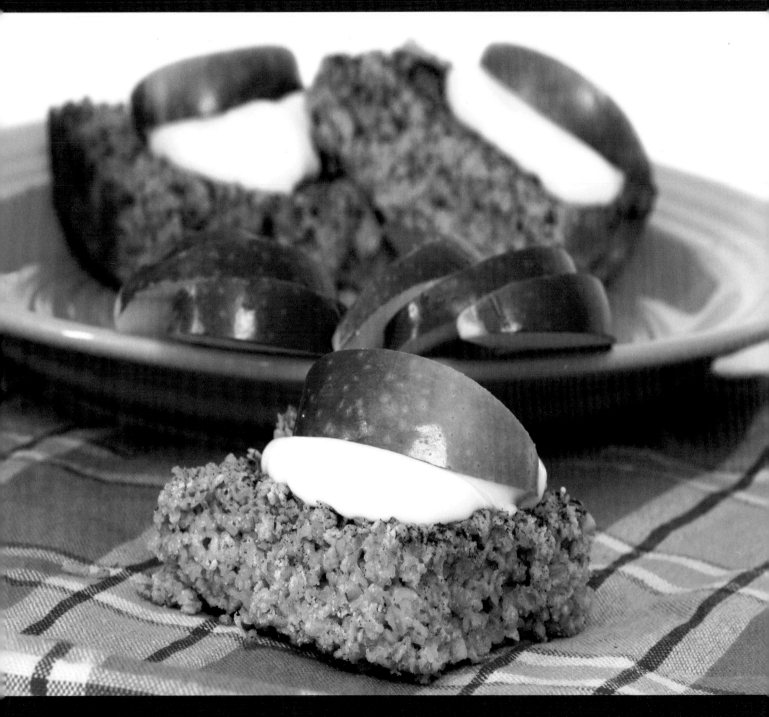

BAKED OATMEAL SQUARES

ontains carbohydrates and protein but I tend to have additional protein such as scrambled egg whites or mini quiche (see mini quiche recipe) with these.

Can be made ahead of time and kept in fridge for up to 4 days for meal times.

- ▶ 2 ½ cups of skim or unsweetened almond milk
- ▶ 1 cup steel cut oats
- ▶ 1 tsp. of flaxseed oil
- ▶ 1 tsp. of pure vanilla extract
- ▶ Pinch of salt

- ▶ 2 tbsp. of sugar free pancake syrup
- ▶ ½ tsp. each of ground nutmeg & cinnamon
- ▶ 1 ½ cups peeled diced apples
- ▶ 2/3 cup unsweetened raisins (optional)
- ▶ 2 cups egg whites

- ❖ Preheat oven to 375° F.

- ❖ In medium saucepan, heat milk on the stove until hot but not boiling.

- ❖ Stir in oats, flaxseed oil, vanilla extract, salt, syrup, nutmeg, cinnamon and diced apples.

- ❖ Cook just until mixture comes to a boil. Remove from heat, stir in raisins and egg whites.

- ❖ Spray rectangular baking dish with fat free cooking spray and transfer oatmeal mixture to baking dish, cover and bake for 25-30 minutes until liquid is absorbed and oatmeal is creamy. Should puff up a little when finished.

- ❖ Eat immediately or refrigerate, cut into squares and re-heat in microwave.

Optional Garnish: tbsp. of your favorite vanilla low-fat Greek yogurt or sugar free ice cream and a slice of apple!

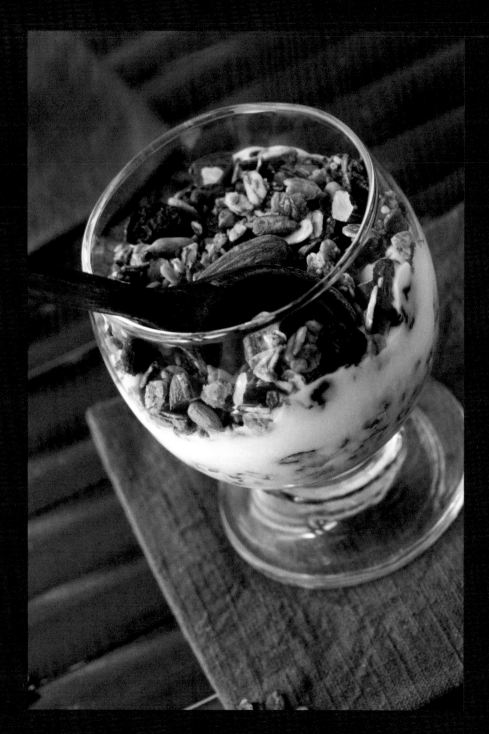

HEALTHY HOMEMADE GRANOLA WITH GREEK YOGURT

This is a meal containing good fats, carbohydrates and protein. Super easy to make granola ahead of time and serve on top of some high protein Greek yogurt in the morning. If you are not having granola with a high protein yogurt then be sure to have with protein such as dry cottage cheese or egg whites to keep blood sugar levels constant as granola is a bit high in natural sugar.

- ▶ 4½ cups of old fashioned oats
- ▶ ½ cup oat bran
- ▶ ½ cup sunflower seeds (I like to use salted to add a little more flavor)
- ▶ ½ cup raw almonds
- ▶ ¼ cup raw cashews
- ▶ ¼ cup chopped pecans

- ▶ ½ cup olive oil
- ▶ 2 tsp. cinnamon
- ▶ ½ cup of sugar free pancake syrup
- ▶ 2 tbsp. of barley malt or molasses
- ▶ ¼ cup boiling water
- ▶ 1 cup unsweetened raisins, chopped apricots or chopped prunes

- ❖ Preheat oven to 275° F and place rack in middle position.
- ❖ In large mixing bowl combine oats, oat bran, sunflower seeds & nuts.
- ❖ Using separate bowl combine oil, cinnamon, syrup, boiling water and barley malt or molasses. Stir into oat mixture.
- ❖ Toss to coat evenly and spread granola evenly on cookie sheet, squeeze little clumps together with your hands to make clusters (spray with olive oil cooking spray).
- ❖ Bake 25-30 minutes
- ❖ Add dried fruit and bake another 5-15 minutes until very slightly golden brown.
- ❖ Cool - can store in air tight container for 1-2 weeks.

Place ½-1 cup of high protein Greek yogurt in a bowl and top with ½ cup of granola.

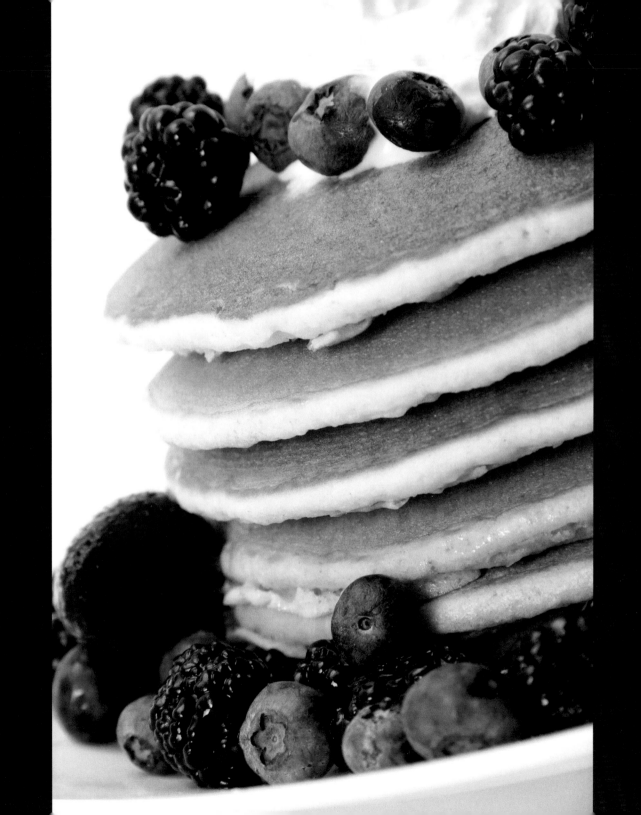

PROTEIN PANCAKES

*T*hese are a complete meal, have 1-3 of them for any meal depending on your activity and personal goals. Top with sugar free pancake syrup or I like to use a tiny bit of fancy molasses.

These freeze very well. You can cool and freeze in freezer bags, remove from freezer and thaw in refrigerator for up to one week. You can re-heat in microwave or toaster when ready to eat.

- ▶ 3 ½ cups of unsweetened applesauce
- ▶ 1 cups old fashioned oats
- ▶ ½ cup spelt or favorite multigrain / gluten free flour
- ▶ 1 cup brown rice flour
- ▶ ¾ cup of 1 % or dry cottage cheese whipped in blender with 3 tbsp. oil & 1 ½ cups of egg whites

- ▶ 2 tsp. baking powder
- ▶ ½ cup of vanilla flavored or plain protein powder (I use the ISO PRO Low Carb or Iso Natural Powder)
- ▶ Cinnamon to taste

- ❖ Add all ingredients together, stir until combined.

- ❖ Heat a grill or non-stick frying pan, spray with cooking spray.

- ❖ Using a 1/3 cup measure, pour pancakes on grill.

- ❖ Serve immediately or cool & refrigerate up to 1 week or put in freezer bags to freeze for later!

Can also double or triple this recipe so you always have lots on hand.

Optional Garnish: Top with a few fresh berries and a tbsp. of fat free cool whip or vanilla yogurt. Could also use a tbsp of diabetic or low calorie pancake syrup if you wish.

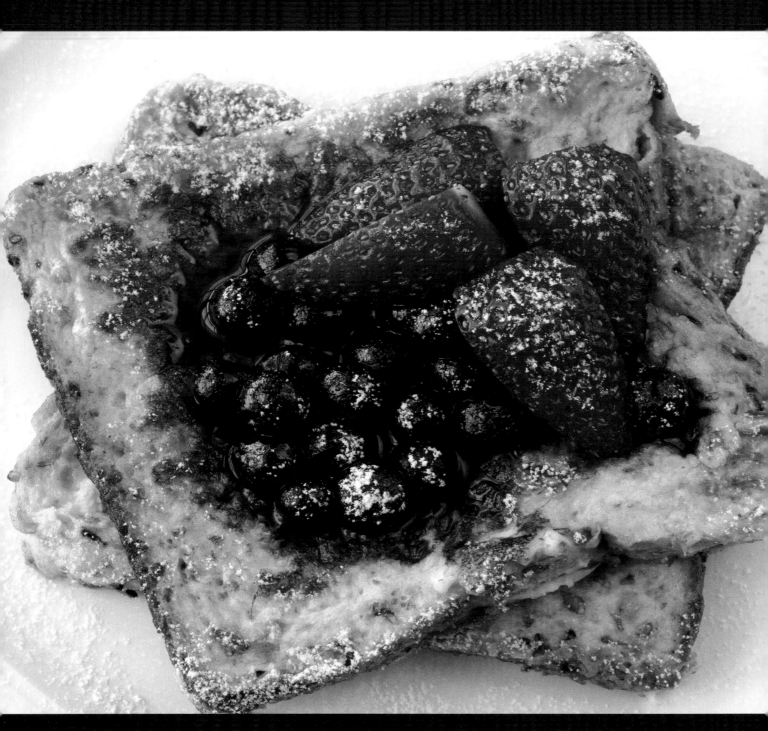

HEALTHY FRENCH TOAST

*T*his recipe offers some protein but it's a good idea to have a little extra protein with this such as scrambled egg whites, mini quiche or some high protein Greek yogurt. One to three pieces of French toast would be a serving depending on gender and activity level.

- ▶ **2 pieces of flour free bread made with sprouted grains**

- ▶ **3 egg whites**

- ▶ **Cinnamon to taste**

- ❖ Mix egg whites and cinnamon together.

- ❖ Soak each piece of bread in egg whites until thoroughly soaked up on both sides.

- ❖ Spray pan or grill with cooking spray and cook each piece of toast until golden brown on both sides.

- ❖ Top with sugar free pancake syrup and a few fresh sliced strawberries.

Optional Garnish: Heat 1 cup of berries such as blueberries or huckleberries on stove top with a ¼ cup (or less) of water and reduce berries to create a berry sauce. Top your French toast with a tbsp. of cooked berries & sauce along with a few slices of fresh strawberries and a pinch of Splenda. You could also use tbsp. of all natural maple syrup or diabetic pancake syrup.

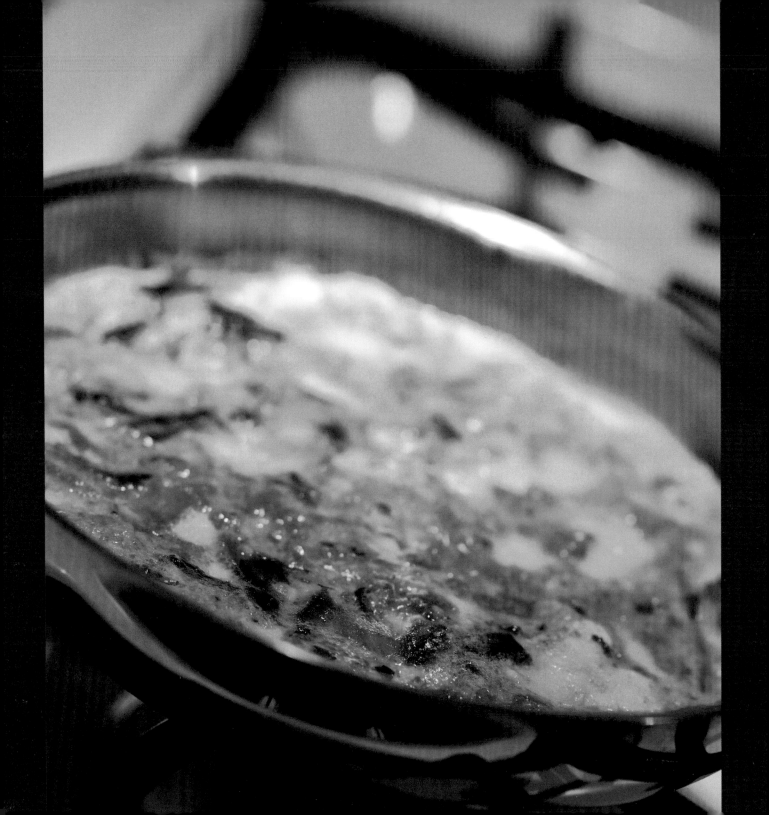

SPICY EGG OMELETE

*T*his is a single serving, you could use less egg white or more depending on appetite… adjust veggies according to taste

- ► 6-8 egg whites, I usually buy the natural liquid ones without any additives

- ► 1 tbsp. of olive oil

- ► ¼ cup sliced banana peppers

- ► ½ small yellow onion – thinly sliced

- ► 1 cup fresh chopped spinach

- ► ½ fresh tomato – thinly sliced and cut lengthwise

- ► 2 tbsp. shredded no-fat cheese

- ► Salt & Pepper to taste

- ❖ Sauté all ingredients except egg whites and low fat cheese in small frying pan until veggies are tender and juices are soaked up. Remove from pan and set aside.

- ❖ Spray frying pan with no-fat cooking spray, add egg whites. When the egg whites start to form on the bottom, add veggies that had been set aside back into pan on top of the egg whites.

- ❖ Cover and cook until omelet is almost done and fluffy. Remove lid, add no-fat cheese and cook 1 minute more. Remove from pan and serve immediately.

SPICY SPINACH MINI QUICHE

*T*his is a protein and should be eaten with one of the carbohydrate choices such as the baked oatmeal squares found on page 29.

- ► 1 red pepper, sliced thinly
- ► 1 red onion, sliced thinly
- ► 1 cup chopped fresh spinach
- ► 5 fresh mushrooms, sliced very thin
- ► 1 jalapeno pepper sliced thin (optional)
- ► 1 tbsp. of olive oil

- ► Few dashes of hot sauce (optional)
- ► 1 ½ cups shredded fat free skim cheddar or mozzarella cheese (high in protein)
- ► 2 cups egg whites
- ► salt and pepper to taste

- ❖ Sauté all veggies in the olive oil.
- ❖ Remove from heat and add salt and pepper.
- ❖ Put about 1-2 tbsp. of veggie mixture in the bottom of sprayed muffin tins.
- ❖ Top with egg whites, about 2 per tin.
- ❖ Dash with hot sauce and then sprinkle fat free shredded cheese on top of each one.
- ❖ Bake at 350° F for 12-18 minutes until desired firmness.

EGG MCHEALTHINS

*T*his is a complete meal offering carbohydrates, protein and good fats. Have one or two sandwiches depending on gender and activity level.

▶ **2 slim brown rice cakes or corn thins (these are ½ the width of regular ones)**

▶ **4 egg whites**

▶ **30 grams (few thin slices) of fat free skim mozzarella or cheddar**

▶ **2 oz. of low sodium, pre-cooked, fat free ham**

❖ Spray frying pan with no-stick cooking spray and fry egg whites over medium-low heat. Don't scramble, just cook whole and flip like a fried egg.

❖ When the egg whites are almost done cooking, turn heat to low and top with sliced cheese and ham.

❖ Cover till cheese is melted and ham is warm.

❖ Spread a thin layer of deodorized coconut oil or mashed avocado on to each rice cake.

❖ Place egg/cheese/ham between two rice cakes like a sandwich and enjoy!

PROTEIN PACKED BOWLS

*D*on't like cottage cheese? Have you ever tried the dry cottage cheese? It is similar to a feta cheese consistency, very versatile, packed with protein and can be used in almost anything. The dry is also fat free. You can whip it, cook it (it doesn't melt easily), freeze it or use it in place of feta cheese. Try one of these sweet bowls to see what you think. If you like wet cottage cheese, you can use the 1% which is still fairly high in protein but be aware that the wet stuff is extremely high in sodium as well.

Combine all ingredients in a bowl and enjoy!

Apple Pie Bowl

- ► 1 cup dry cottage cheese
- ► ¾ cup unsweetened applesauce
- ► 1 small diced apple
- ► Cinnamon and Splenda or other sugar substitute to taste

Rhubarb Pie Bowl

- ► 1 cup dry cottage cheese
- ► ¾ cup to 1 cup of stewed rhubarb
- ► Cinnamon and Splenda or other sugar substitute to taste

Pumpkin Pie Bowl

- ► 1 cup dry cottage cheese (I like to use ½ 1% for this bowl as it can be a bit dry)
- ► 1 cup pure pumpkin puree
- ► 2 tbsp. unsweetened raisins
- ► Cinnamon and Splenda or other sugar substitute to taste.

PROTEIN ENERGY BARS

*T*hese are a complete meal offering carbohydrates, protein and healthy fats. Great for breakfast when you're in a hurry or on-the-go.

- ► 3 cups old fashioned oats

- ► 3 cups crisp brown rice (can find at a health food store)

- ► 1 ½ cups all natural peanut butter

- ► 1 ½ cups unsweetened apple sauce

- ► 1 cup Carr's or other diabetic pancake syrup (can find in most pharmacies-food section)

- ► ½ cup Splenda or sugar substitute

- ► 1 ½ cups of chopped prunes or dried apricots or combination

- ► 6 scoops (1 cup) of vanilla protein powder.

- ❖ Melt peanut butter in pan, remove from heat and add all other ingredients.

- ❖ Line a clean square pan with parchment paper, transfer and press mixture into this pan… I use parchment paper on top to press down as this is a sticky mixture. Keep parchment paper on top while freezing

- ❖ Freeze for 2-3 hours, remove from freezer and cut into squares.

I store mine in the freezer and eat them frozen, they are very yummy cold. If they're a bit hard, just thaw for 2 minutes before eating.

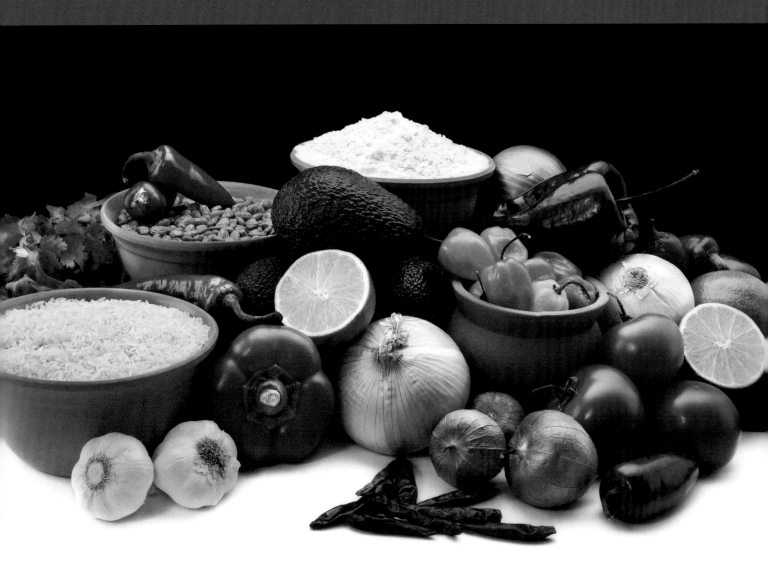

Recipe's for LEAN Lunch & Dinners

Options for meals 3,4 & 5 of the day

- ❖ Tuna & Avocado Open Face Sandwich........................36
- ❖ Easy Rice & Salsa Protein Bowl.....37
- ❖ Buffalo Chicken Strips with Avocado Coleslaw........................39
- ❖ Grilled Chicken Tacos 41
- ❖ Easy Fish Tacos with Spicy Mango Salsa 42
- ❖ Asian Inspired Chicken Lettuce Wraps....................45
- ❖ Thai Chicken Salad with Peanut Dressing 46
- ❖ Chicken Quinoa Salad............49
- ❖ Shrimp Rice Rolls.................51
- ❖ Super Lean Chili 53
- ❖ Mexican Pot Pie 54
- ❖ Taco Soup 56
- ❖ Mock Spaghetti Bowl............57
- ❖ Peppered Steak and Rice Plate.....61
- ❖ Guilt Free German Meatloaf........63
- ❖ Lean Mean Meatballs in Port Reduction 65
- ❖ Spinach Chicken Bowl.............66
- ❖ Cranberry Chutney Chicken........67
- ❖ Cabbage Lentil Stew 69
- ❖ Curry Chicken & Rice Dish 71
- ❖ Halibut In Wine & Fig Marinade.....73
- ❖ Wasabi Maple Salmon.............75
- ❖ BBQ Chili, Lime & Beer Chicken with Mango Salsa..................77
- ❖ Fresh Mango Salsa 81
- ❖ Stir Fry Rice 83
- ❖ Chicken & Cashews with Rice Noodles....................85
- ❖ Shrimp & Scallops In Wine Reduction 87

TUNA & AVOCADO OPEN FACE SANDWICH

*T*his is a meal with all 3 macronutrients; carbs, protein and healthy fat. If you're not overly carb conscious or if you are very active, you may substitute the rice cakes for sprouted grain bread but this is very tasty with the rice cakes.

- ▶ 2 rice cakes or two pieces of squirrely bread

- ▶ 1 can of tuna packed in water and drained

- ▶ ½ mashed avocado

- ▶ 2-3 chopped green onions

- ▶ 2 chopped dill pickles with a little of the juice or I like to use the bread and butter pickles

- ▶ ¼ cup high protein Greek yogurt

- ▶ ½ celery stalk (diced very small)

- ▶ 2 tbsp. jar sliced peppers such as banana peppers or sliced jalapenos

- ❖ Combine all ingredients except rice cakes into bowl.

- ❖ Mix thoroughly and spread ½ the mixture on each rice cake or slice of bread.

EASY RICE & SALSA PROTEIN BOWL

his recipe contains both carbohydrates & protein, makes a good meal or easy snack.

- ▶ 1 cup cooked brown rice
- ▶ 1 cup dry cottage cheese
- ▶ ½ - 1 cup of your favorite salsa

- ▶ ¼ cup of chopped veggies such as water chestnuts, banana peppers & green onion (if you like some crunch in the mix)

- ❖ Combine all ingredients in a bowl and eat cold or heat for 30 seconds in microwave to warm.

This very simple dish is surprisingly tasty and very easy if you have cooked rice in the fridge.

Inspired by my girlfriend Carrie!

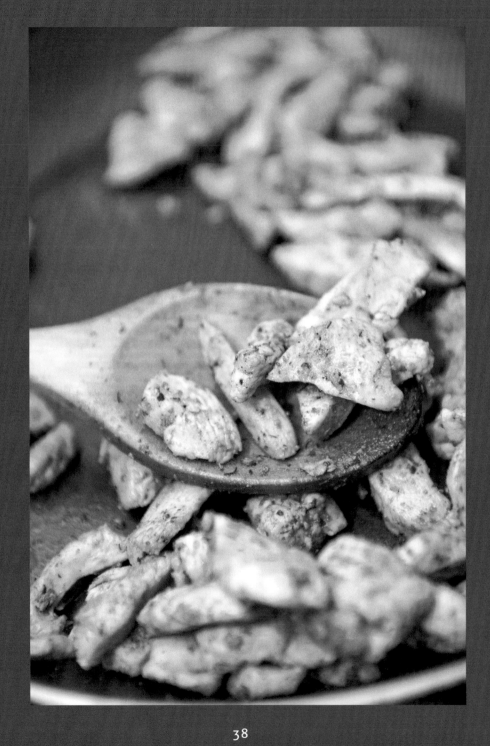

BUFFALO CHICKEN STRIPS WITH AVOCADO COLESLAW

*T*his is a great meal that is simple to prepare and offers both protein and carbohydrates in the form of veggies.

Buffalo chicken strips

- ► 3-4 boneless skinless chicken breasts - sliced into strips

- ► buffalo hot sauce to coat chicken (lots of varieties that are only 5 calories per tsp.)

- ❖ Sauté chicken in a tiny bit of olive oil or bake in oven until done. Remove from heat and coat with Buffalo Sauce.

Avocado coleslaw

- ► 2 cups each of shredded green and red cabbage
- ► 1 cup shredded carrots
- ► 5-6 chopped green onions
- ► ½ cup shredded celery
- ► 1 shredded jalapeno pepper (seeds removed)
- ► 2 tbsp. balsamic vinegar

- ► ½ cup no-fat Greek yogurt
- ► 1 tbsp. Brown Sugar Splenda
- ► 1 tbsp. each of olive oil & hot sauce
- ► Juice from ½ lime
- ► 1 tsp. each of pepper & dry mustard powder
- ► 1 avocado, peeled and mashed
- ► ½ cup chopped cilantro

- ❖ Mix all veggies for coleslaw together, except avocado and cilantro.
- ❖ In separate bowl, mix vinegar, yogurt, Splenda, oil, lime, spices & hot sauce together
- ❖ Add to veggies.
- ❖ Before serving… add mashed avocado and cilantro. Combine well
- ❖ Dish some of the buffalo chicken strips onto a plate along with some avocado coleslaw

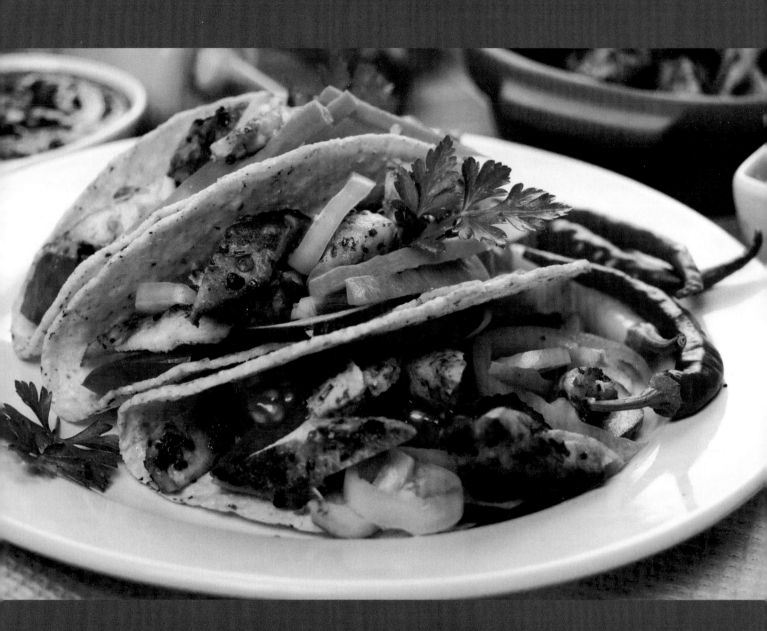

GRILLED CHICKEN TACOS

Tacos

- ► 1 lb. boneless, skinless chicken breast cut into thin strips
- ► 1 tbsp. of chili powder
- ► ½ tsp. each of cumin and pepper
- ► 1 tbsp. lime juice
- ► 1 tbsp. of olive oil

- ► 1 small diced onion
- ► ¼ cup water
- ► taco shells or homemade corn tortillas from corn mesa flour (found in most grocery stores in Mexican section or by cornmeal). Prepare per package instructions.

Toppings

- ► lettuce
- ► chopped tomatoes
- ► low or fat free shredded cheese
- ► banana peppers

- ► sliced cucumbers
- ► salsa
- ► guacamole

- ❖ Sauté chicken, oil, chili powder, cumin, pepper, lime juice and onion until chicken is cooked thoroughly.

- ❖ Add water and simmer on med-low heat for another 15-20 minutes.

- ❖ Heat taco shells or prepare homemade corn tortillas with corn mesa flour as per package directions.

- ❖ Add 2 oz. of cooked chicken to each taco shell or tortilla and toppings as desired.

- ❖ Serve with Salsa and 1 tbsp. of homemade guacamole.

EASY FISH TACOS WITH SPICY MANGO SALSA

Mango Salsa – can be made ahead of time and refrigerated for up to 2 days.

- ▶ 2 mangos
- ▶ one red onion
- ▶ 2 peppers, yellow, orange or red
- ▶ 1 fresh jalapeno pepper
- ▶ 1 can water chestnuts

- ▶ ½ cup chopped cilantro
- ▶ Juice of one lime
- ▶ 1 tbsp. of chili powder
- ▶ ½ tsp each of salt, cumin, pepper
- ▶ ½ cup chopped cilantro

- ❖ Dice first 5 ingredients together in bowl.
- ❖ Add rest of ingredients, toss and refrigerate until ready to use. Salsa will last for up to two days in refrigerator.

Corn Tortilla's

Use soft all-corn tortillas (small ones) or homemade corn mesa tortilla's – about 6" diameter. Can buy authentic corn mesa flour in most grocery stores – prepare as per package directions just before preparing fish and keep warm on lowest heat in oven until fish filling is ready.

Fish Filling

- ► 1lb. of white fish such as halibut, cod or basa

- ► 1 tbsp. olive oil

- ► 1 tbsp. each of lime and lemon juice

- ► ½ tsp. each of cumin, coriander and pepper

- ► 1 tbsp. hot sauce

- ❖ Sauté all ingredients together until fish is thoroughly cooked and keep warm on stovetop until ready to serve, if mixture seems too dry, add a little water.

Toppings

- ► 1 cucumber – thinly sliced

- ► 1 avocado – chopped or homemade guacamole

- ❖ Fill tortillas with 2 oz. of fish filling, top with mango salsa, thinly sliced cucumber and 1 tbsp. of chopped avocado or homemade guacamole. Fold in half and enjoy!

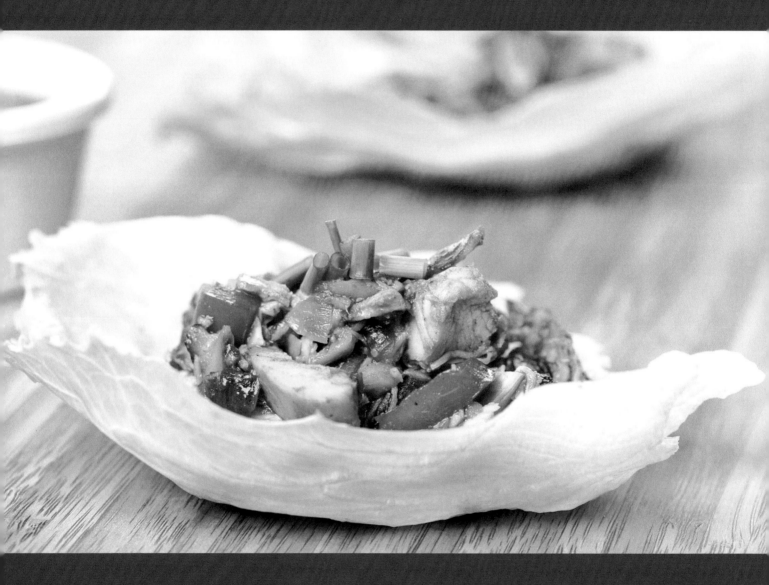

ASIAN INSPIRED CHICKEN LETTUCE WRAPS

- ► 1 lb. diced boneless skinless chicken breast
- ► 1 tbsp. olive oil
- ► 1 tbsp. Asian five spice or 1 tbsp. equal amounts of a mixture of fennel, cloves, allspice, pepper and cayenne
- ► 2 tbsp. minced ginger
- ► 2 tbsp. minced garlic
- ► 1 small red onion – diced
- ► 2 tbsp. tamari or low sodium soy sauce

- ► 2 tbsp. all natural peanut butter
- ► ½ cup low sodium organic chicken broth
- ► 1 tbsp. fancy molasses
- ► 4 green onions or chives
- ► 6-8 sliced fresh mushrooms
- ► 1 cup shredded carrots
- ► 1 cup bean sprouts
- ► ½ cup chopped water chestnuts
- ► 1-2 heads of large leaf lettuce

❖ Sauté chicken in olive oil over high heat until chicken is cooked thoroughly.

❖ Add remaining ingredients, except lettuce, and simmer over medium low heat until liquid is absorbed and mixture thickens. Can add more chicken broth if mixture seems too dry…. should be a light sauce on mixture. Keep warm on stovetop over low heat until ready to use

❖ Wash and pat large lettuce leaves dry and place on serving dish. Put chicken mixture in another serving dish.

❖ To serve, wrap approx. ½ cup of chicken mixture in a large lettuce leaf. Fold in half and eat like a taco or fold up like a roll.

Optional Garnish: Chopped green onions or chives and chopped Roma tomatoes.

THAI CHICKEN SALAD WITH PEANUT DRESSING

Peanut Dressing - Can be made ahead of time and refrigerated for up to one week.

- ▶ ¼ cup of rice vinegar
- ▶ 2 tbsp. sesame oil
- ▶ ¼ cup of all natural peanut butter
- ▶ 2 tbsp. tamari or low sodium soy sauce

- ▶ 2 tbsp. fancy molasses (optional)
- ▶ 1 tbsp each of minced ginger and garlic
- ▶ 4 tbsp. of brown sugar or sugar substitute. I like to use Brown Sugar Splenda

- ❖ Place all ingredients in a blender and blend until smooth.

Prepare Chicken:

- ▶ 1 lb. of boneless, skinless chicken breast cut into short strips
- ▶ 1 tbsp. olive or sesame oil

- ▶ 1 tbsp. of tamari or low sodium soy sauce

- ❖ Sauté these three ingredients together on medium-high heat until chicken is thoroughly cooked and set aside to cool, while preparing salad

Prepare Salad:

1 head of your favorite lettuce. I like to use romaine. Wash, dry, cut into pieces and divide/assemble onto serving plates. Top each dish of lettuce with the following:

- ▶ ¼ cup shredded purple cabbage
- ▶ ¼ cup raw bean sprouts
- ▶ ¼ cup shredded or julienne carrots
- ▶ ¼ cup sliced fresh mushrooms

- ▶ 2 tbsp. chopped green onion or chives
- ▶ 2 tbsp. unsweetened coconut (optional)
- ▶ 2 tbsp. chopped cilantro

- ❖ Place cooled chicken on top of each plate of salad and drizzle with desired amount of dressing. Enjoy.

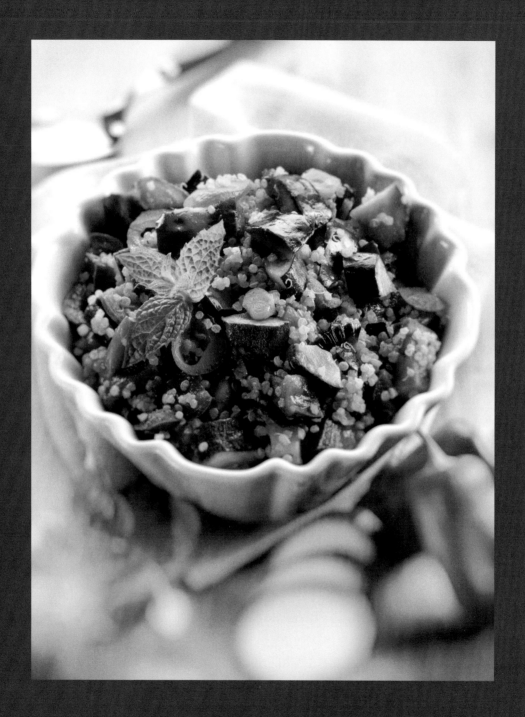

CHICKEN QUINOA SALAD

Prepare Chicken:

- ► 1 lb. of boneless, skinless chicken breast cut into short strips
- ► 1 tbsp. olive or sesame oil
- ❖ Sautee these three ingredients together until chicken is fully cooked and set aside to cool while preparing salad

- ► 1 tbsp. of tamari or low sodium soy sauce

Prepare Quinoa:

- ► 1 cup rinsed quinoa

- ► 2 cups low sodium chicken broth

- ❖ In medium pot, bring quinoa and chicken broth to a boil. Cover and reduce heat to medium low. Simmer for 15-20 minutes, fluff up with a fork and set aside to cool.

Prepare rest of Salad:

- ► 2 medium cooked yams, diced into little bite size pieces
- ► 1 large onion, diced
- ► 3 garlic cloves, minced
- ► 1 large red bell pepper, diced
- ► 1 medium zucchini, diced
- ► ½ small head purple cabbage, shredded

- ► 1 tsp. ground coriander seed
- ► 1 tbsp. fresh squeezed lemon juice
- ► 1 tsp. lime juice
- ► 1 tbsp. Tamari or low-sodium soy sauce
- ► 1 tsp. of chili powder
- ► 1 tbsp. fancy molasses or pure maple syrup
- ► ½ cup chopped cilantro

- ❖ Combine cooked chicken, quinoa and salad mixture. Mix well and enjoy immediately!

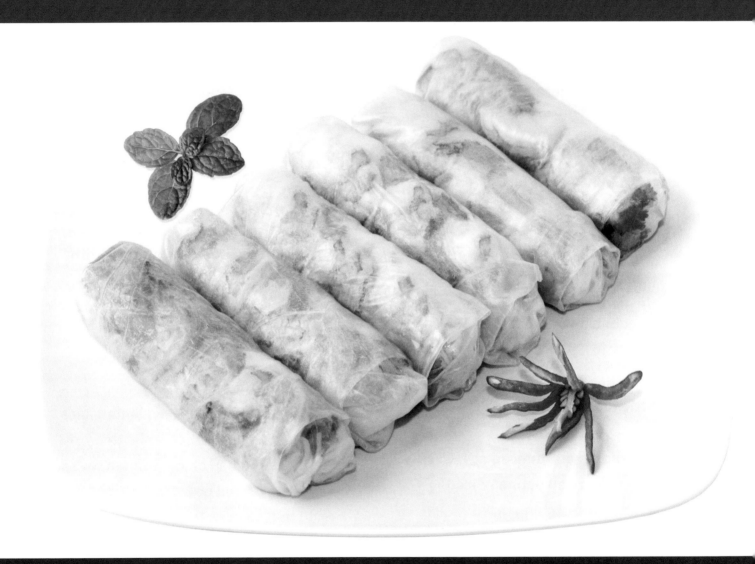

SHRIMP RICE ROLLS

- ❖ Sauté 1 lb. of small to medium peeled & deveined shrimp (with tails off) until cooked thoroughly
- ❖ Prepare one package of thin rice noodles as per package directions, drain and coat with 2 tbsp. of sesame oil and a tsp. of salt – toss noodles and set aside to cool

<u>Prepare rest of ingredients in separate dishes:</u>

- ▶ **2 cucumbers, sliced julienne style – slice a cucumber lengthwise in tiny strips with the peel on. Discard center of cucumber (seeds).**
- ▶ **2 carrots: sliced julienne style - slice carrots lengthwise into tiny sticks**

- ▶ **1 bunch fresh chopped cilantro**
- ▶ **1 head iceberg or other lettuce – wash & pat dry, cut into pieces.**
- ▶ **2 bunches green onions**

- ❖ Get Rice Paper (also known as rice wraps) ready! Use two large plates with edges (or you can use a shallow dish), fill with very warm water about 3" deep.
- ❖ Soak rice wraps in warm water for about one minute covering all edges until soft and flexible.
- ❖ Remove wrap from water, shake off excess water and lay flat on cutting board. Have another one soaking while making first wrap and continue like this so you always have a rice wrap ready to be filled until all are assembled.
- ❖ Start to assemble rice wrap by filling one half with some rice noodles, 3-4 cooked shrimp, few sticks each of carrot, cucumber, lettuce, cilantro and green onions.
- ❖ Starting at one edge of wrap, roll wrap until all filling is wrapped into nice neat roll tucking in edges as you go.
- ❖ Set prepared wraps on parchment paper and cover with plastic wrap until ready to eat. Can be refrigerated for 12 hours.

Serve with dipping sauce such as hot chili Thai sauce, peanut dressing from page 54, or fish sauce.

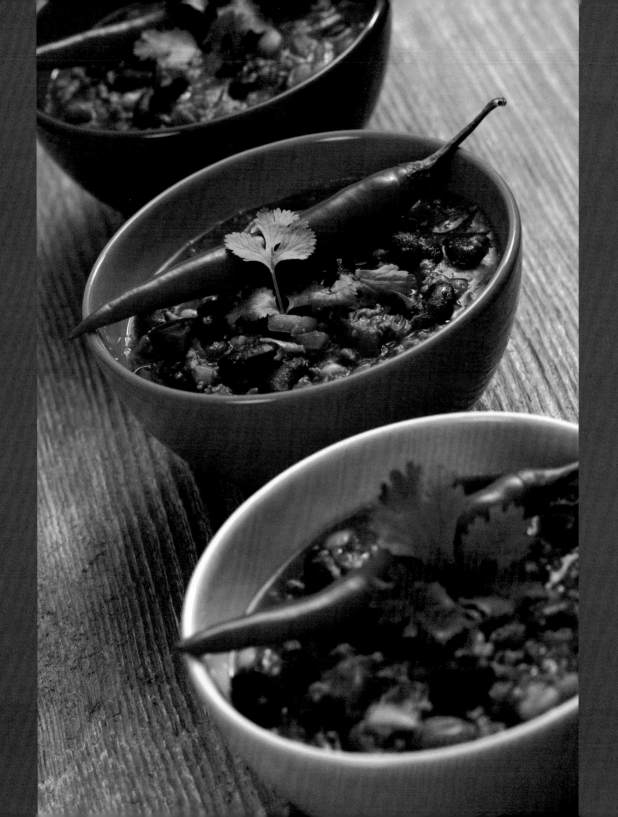

SUPER LEAN CHILI

- ▶ Sauté 1lb. of ground chicken or turkey breast meat in 1 tbsp. of olive oil for 5 min over medium heat.

- ▶ Add 1 cup each of diced mushrooms, diced zucchini, diced onions, diced carrots, diced celery, 2 cups finely shredded cabbage and three minced garlic cloves

- ▶ Sauté meat and veggies together over medium low heat until all veggies are tender, about another 5-7minutes.

- ▶ Add 1 can (796ml) of diced tomatoes in juice

- ▶ Add 1 small can of tomato paste

- ▶ Rinse and drain 1 (796ml) can each of white kidney beans, red kidney beans and black beans… add to meat and veggies

- ▶ Add two cups of veggie juice such as V8

- ▶ Add ½ cup of fancy molasses

- ▶ Add 1 cup of frozen corn

- ▶ Add desired spice to taste: chili powder, salt, pepper, cayenne, etc…

- ❖ Simmer covered for 45minutes over low heat

- ❖ Remove cover and simmer another 15minutes.

Optional Garnish: Garnish with a fresh pepper of your choice and some chopped cilantro

MEXICAN POT PIE

Prepare corn crust

- ▶ **1 1/2 cups of corn mesa flour**
- ▶ **½ cup cornmeal**
- ▶ **¼ cup olive oil**

- ▶ **2 cups water**
- ▶ **2 tsp. salt**

- ❖ Add all ingredients together

- ❖ Mix and roll out onto cutting board into large rectangular or square shape to match baking dish that you will be using

- ❖ Roll dough out to ¼" thickness and larger than pan so crust will cover sides.

- ❖ Place pan upside down over rolled dough.

- ❖ Flip cutting board and baking dish over so dough is laying in baking dish.

- ❖ Press into dish covering bottom and sides of pan. This dough pieces together easily if you have tears or not enough to cover sides.

Prepare filling

- 1 cup each of no fat shredded mozza. And cheddar cheese
- Sautee 1 lb. of ground turkey or chicken breast meat until thoroughly cooked (you can substitute ground meat for dry cottage cheese if preferred which does not have to be pre-cooked). Add to large bowl with remaining ingredients [except cheese]:

- 5 cups of prepared rice – brown, wild or rice of choice
- 1 cup of your favorite salsa
- 2 cans of rinsed and drained beans
- ½ cup feta cheese
- 1 can (500ml) of diced tomatoes with juice
- ½ cup veggie juice such as V8

❖ Put ½ of the filling into corn crust, sprinkle with 1 cup no fat shredded mozzarella and cheddar cheeses. Place rest of filling in pan, top with another cup of no fat cheese.

❖ Bake at 350° F for 45 minutes

❖ Serve with homemade guacamole and no fat Greek yogurt if desired.

TACO SOUP

- 4-5 boneless skinless chicken breast
- 1 tbsp. of organic chicken base
- ½ cup salsa of choice
- 1 can tomato paste
- 1 large can diced tomatoes
- 2 fresh diced tomatoes
- 1 onion - diced
- 3 stalks of celery – diced
- ½ large head of cabbage – finely shredded
- 1 large can of drained and rinsed black beans
- Spices as desired: salt, pepper, chili powder, garlic powder
- 1 cup of Greek no-fat yogurt
- 1 avocado- Sliced
- Fresh chopped cilantro

❖ Boil chicken breasts in large pot of water (approximately 3 liters).

❖ Remove chicken breast once fully cooked and shred with two forks into bite size pieces.

❖ Add rest of ingredients to chicken broth.

❖ Add cooked shredded chicken and simmer on medium-low heat until all veggies are tender. About 45minutes.

❖ Top with 1 tbsp. of Greek yogurt, slice of avocado and chopped fresh cilantro

MOCK SPAGHETTI BOWL

- ► 1 large spaghetti squash
- ► 1 lb. ground chicken or turkey breast meat
- ► 3 tbsp. olive oil
- ► 1 large onion - dices
- ► 2 red peppers – diced
- ► 2 stalks of celery – diced
- ► 10 medium fresh mushrooms – diced

- ► 1 fresh zucchini - diced
- ► 2 fresh tomatoes – chopped
- ► 3 cloves of garlic – minced
- ► 1 can tomato paste
- ► 1 large can diced tomatoes and juice
- ► 1 tbsp. Splenda (optional)
- ► Spices to taste: salt, pepper, cayenne

- ❖ Slice squash in half lengthwise, remove seeds with spoon and all stringy parts with a fork. Place face down on baking sheet lined with parchment paper and bake for 45-60minutes on 350° F until tender. While squash is cooking, prepare sauce;

- ❖ Sauce: Sauté chicken or turkey breast meat in olive oil until cooked thoroughly… approx. 10 minutes

- ❖ Add all diced veggies except tomatoes. Sauté until tender.

- ❖ Add tomato paste, diced canned tomatoes with juice and spices.

- ❖ Simmer covered on low for 40 minutes or until thickened.

❖ When squash is tender and cooked, remove from oven and cool slightly so you can handle. Using a fork, remove squash away from the skin of the squash so that it resembles spaghetti noodles. Place back into squash skin to use as a bowl or onto a plate if you wish.

❖ Top with prepared sauce and a few tbsp. of shredded no fat cheese if you like.

Spaghetti squash can also be substituted for brown rice or kamut spaghetti noodles if you would like the extra carbohydrates and/or don't mind the carbs! You can also substitute the ground meat for dry cottage cheese which is very high protein and no fat. If doing this, skip step 2 and add cottage cheese at the end – after Step 5.

Remember...Every time you eat is an opportunity to nourish your body.

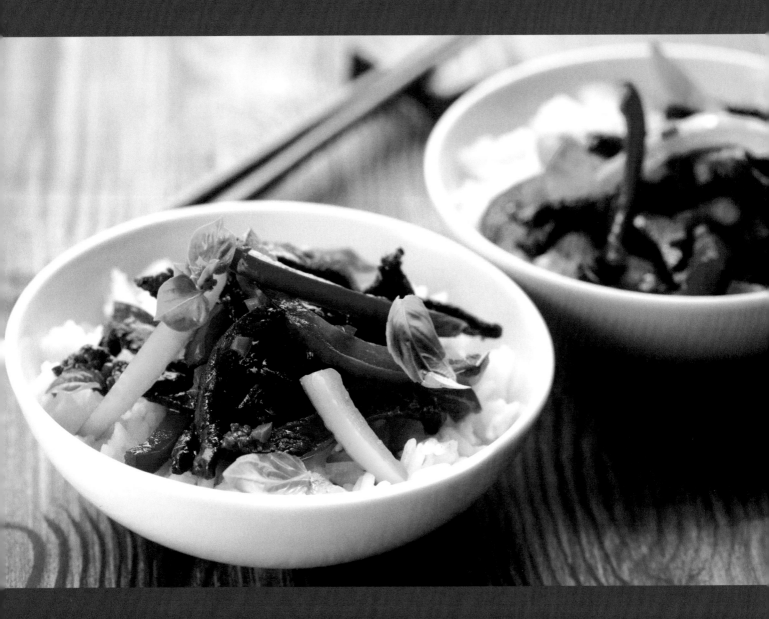

PEPPERED STEAK AND RICE PLATE

- ► 2 lbs. of lean beef such as round steak – sliced into thin strips
- ► 3 tbsp. of tomato paste
- ► ¼ cup red wine
- ► 2 tbsp. olive oil
- ► 2 fresh colored peppers – sliced thinly
- ► 1 large onion – sliced thinly
- ► 2 stalks of celery – sliced into strips

- ► 2 cloves of garlic
- ► 1 fresh jalapeno – seeds removed if you don't like too spicy – diced
- ► 2 tbsp. of minced ginger
- ► 3 tbsp. of low sodium soy sauce
- ► 1 tbsp. of Brown Sugar Splenda
- ► Pepper and spices to taste
- ► 4 cups of rice – prepared per package directions

- ❖ Season beef with salt and pepper as desired. Place sliced beef in crock pot on high with tomato paste and red wine.

- ❖ Cook beef in crock pot for approx. 2 hours or until beef is cooked and tender

- ❖ In separate medium size frying pan, sauté all veggies in olive oil until tender but not overcooked. Add soy sauce and Brown Sugar Splenda, stir until combined.

- ❖ Add veggies to crockpot and mix with beef strips.

- ❖ Place serving of rice into bowl and top with some of the beef & veggie mixture.

- ❖ Garnish with fresh mint or parsley if you like. Can also add a few slices of red and yellow peppers for some crunch.

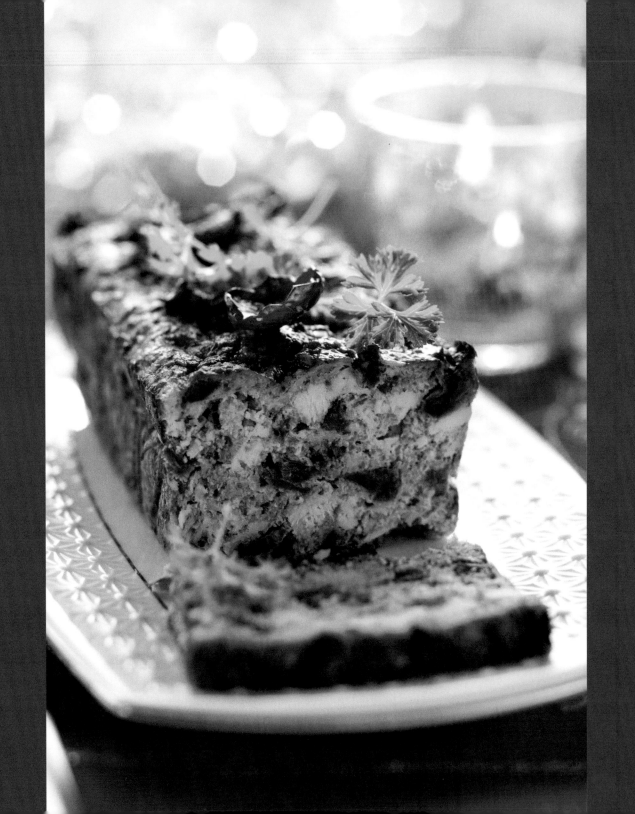

GUILT FREE GERMAN MEATLOAF

- ▶ 1 lb. ground turkey or chicken breast meat
- ▶ 2 cups dry container cottage cheese
- ▶ 1 cup old fashioned oats
- ▶ 1/2 cup egg whites
- ▶ 1 cup drained sauerkraut

- ▶ 2 tbsp. hot horseradish
- ▶ 1 small onion – diced
- ▶ ½ cup diced figs
- ▶ 3 cloves garlic – minced
- ▶ Salt, pepper and cayenne to taste

- ❖ Mix all ingredients together in bowl until well combined.

- ❖ Grease two loaf pans lightly with cooking spray. Press ½ the mixture into each pan or you can use an 8x8 square glass baking dish

- ❖ Bake at 350° F for 45 minutes until thoroughly cooked.

- ❖ Poke knife holes in meatloaf and allow any liquid to seep to top of meatloaf. Can drain excess liquid if needed

- ❖ Bake for an additional 10 minutes. If top gets too brown, loosely cover with tinfoil while baking.

This meal contains carbohydrates and protein so I usually serve with steamed veggies or a tossed green salad. Also like to dip meatloaf in HP sauce, Dijon mustard, or hot sauce.

Optional Garnish: Top with fresh parsley

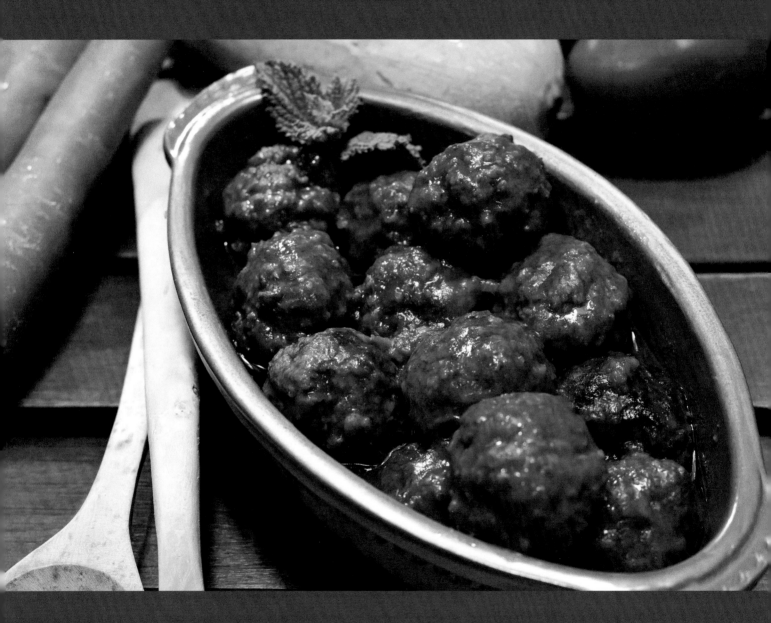

LEAN MEAN MEATBALLS IN PORT REDUCTION

Meatballs

- ▶ 2 lbs. of extra lean ground beef or ground chicken/turkey breast meat
- ▶ 1 cup oats
- ▶ 4 egg whites plus one yolk
- ▶ 1 cup chopped spinach
- ▶ ½ medium onion – diced
- ▶ Salt and pepper to taste

Sauce

- ▶ 1 tbsp. of organic beef base
- ▶ 1 cup water
- ▶ 1 small container of tomato paste
- ▶ ½ cup port wine
- ▶ 2 tbsp. Brown Sugar Splenda
- ▶ 1 tsp. steak spice

- ❖ Mix first 6 ingredients together. Roll into small round balls to form meatballs.
- ❖ Place meatballs in large roasting pan or oven safe baking dish and cook at 350° F for 45 minutes or until thoroughly cooked.
- ❖ Drain excess liquid.
- ❖ While meatballs are cooking, prepare sauce. Add all sauce ingredients together in saucepan. Bring to a boil, stir and lower heat to medium-low. Simmer for about 10-15minutes until thickened.
- ❖ Pour sauce over cooked meatballs coating all.
- ❖ Place meatballs back into oven for another 7-10 minutes until sauce is glazed.

Serve with rice and a steamed veggies!

SPINACH CHICKEN BOWL

Prepare Chicken

- **3-4 boneless skinless chicken breasts**

Boil chicken in boiling water until thoroughly cooked and chicken pulls apart easily. Remove chicken from boiling water using a slotted spoon, place on a plate and let cool. Once cooled, shred chicken using two forks. Set aside while preparing filling and drizzle.

Filling

- 1 medium onion - diced
- 3 cloves of garlic - minced
- 2 tbsp. of olive oil
- 10 cups of fresh spinach
- ½ cup light feta cheese

- ½ cup unsweetened cranberries (usually found in health food stores)
- ½ tsp. each of rosemary, parsley and marjoram,
- Salt and pepper to taste

Sweet and tangy yogurt drizzle

- ½ cup no fat greek yogurt
- 2 tbsp. of apple cider or balsamic vinegar
- 2 tbsp. of olive oil

- 8 fresh strawberries
- ¼ cup of Splenda
- 1 tsp. of dry mustard powder

- ❖ Prepare drizzle by blending all ingredients in a blender until smooth and set aside.
- ❖ Prepare filling by heating oil over medium-high heat. Add onion and sauté for 3-5 minutes until cooked.
- ❖ Add spinach and cook until spinach is soft and tender – approximately another 5 minutes
- ❖ Remove from heat. Add feta cheese, shredded cooked chicken, spices and cranberries.

Serve over a portion of rice and top with a few tbsp. of the drizzle

CRANBERRY CHUTNEY CHICKEN

- ► 3 tbsp. of olive oil
- ► 4 large boneless skinless chicken breast cut in half
- ► 2 large onions – thinly sliced
- ► ½ cup water

- ► 1 cup of whole berry cranberry sauce
- ► 2 tbsp. of red wine vinegar
- ► ½ tsp. each of dried thyme and cayenne
- ► Salt and Pepper to taste

- ❖ Heat oil in large frying pan
- ❖ Add chicken breasts and sauté on high for 3-4 minutes until golden brown on outside but not cooked throughout.
- ❖ Remove chicken breasts and set aside
- ❖ Add onion to pan and sauté until soft and golden
- ❖ Add water, cranberry sauce, vinegar, and spices
- ❖ Cook onions in sauce for another 2-3 minutes until sauce starts to thicken slightly
- ❖ Return chicken to pan, reduce heat to medium low and cover.
- ❖ Cook chicken for another 10-15 minutes until cooked thoroughly.

Serve over a portion of rice or with mashed potatoes or yams!

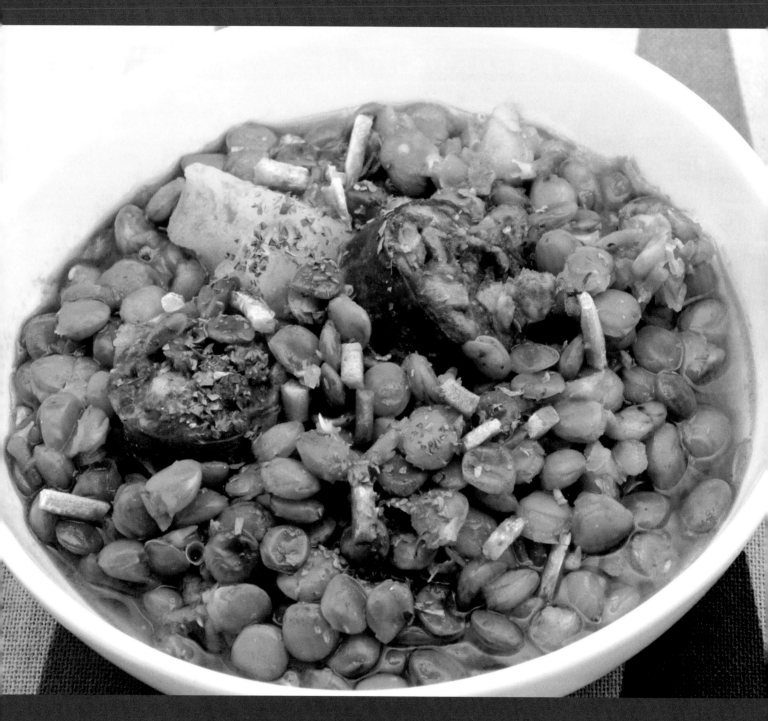

CABBAGE LENTIL STEW

► **4 cups of dried peas/lentils**

Choose variety of yellow/green split peas and lentils (do not use dry beans as cooking time is way longer), cover with water and boil till soft, may need to continue adding a cup of two or water at a time until lentils are fully cooked.

Add:

- ❖ 3 tbsp. of vegetable base (I use all natural stock from jar called Superior Touch Bullion)
- ❖ 1 chopped onion
- ❖ 3-4 cloves garlic
- ❖ 1 chopped zucchini
- ❖ 1 small head of shredded cabbage
- ❖ 1 cup yams – cut into slivers the size of slivered almonds

- ❖ 2 tbsp. of Madras Curry Paste or brand of choice (from jar)
- ❖ ¼ cup fancy molasses
- ❖ Salt and pepper to taste
- ❖ Optional: Add protein - either 2 cups of cooked lean sliced low sodium sausage such as turkey or wild meat sausage or cooked chicken when the rest of the stew is almost cooked.

- ❖ Simmer all ingredients over medium-low heat until cabbage and yams are tender.
- ❖ Remove from heat and stir in 4 tbsp. of no fat greek yogurt.
- ❖ Serve immediately. If not using the optional cooked meat added to the stew, have this meal with a protein such as grilled chicken breast or piece of salmon

Optional Garnish: Top with fresh chopped parsley and a fresh piece of mango or pineapple if you wish

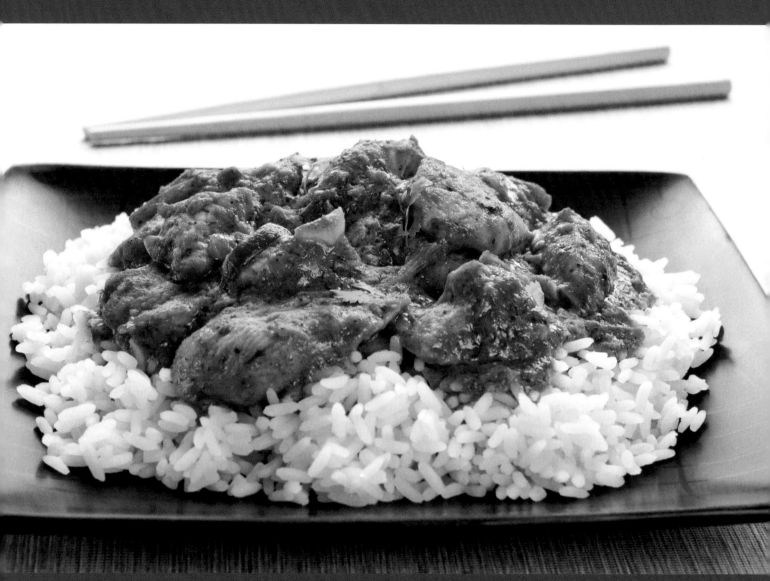

CURRY CHICKEN & RICE DISH

- ▶ 4 boneless skinless chicken breasts – cubed in 1" cubes

- ▶ 2 tbsp. of olive oil

- ▶ 150g package of Indian Madras Meat Curry Paste (found in most grocery stores or you can make up your own curry paste with spices and oil)

- ▶ 1 onion – diced

- ▶ 2 stalks of celery – diced

- ▶ 2 cloves garlic - diced

- ▶ 1 can tomato paste

- ▶ 1 ½ cups plain low fat yogurt or plain Greek yogurt

- ▶ 1 cup unsweetened Coconut Dream milk (60 calories/cup). You could also use light coconut milk if you're not too worried about the few extra calories

- ▶ 1 tbsp. fancy molasses

- ▶ 1 cup frozen peas - optional

- ❖ Sauté chicken in olive oil for approximately 5 minutes.

- ❖ Add packet of Madras Meat Curry Paste, onion, celery and garlic.

- ❖ Sauté on medium-high heat until veggies are tender, approximately 6-7 minutes

- ❖ Remove from heat and add tomato paste, yogurt, coconut milk, fancy molasses and peas. Stir until combined and return to heat.

- ❖ Simmer on medium-low (slow boil) until sauce thickens and chicken is cooked thoroughly - approximately another 20 minutes

You can serve this dish over your favorite rice or if I'm competing I will generally have with a tossed salad as there are already some carbohydrates in this dish.

Garnish with fresh cilantro, yum!!!

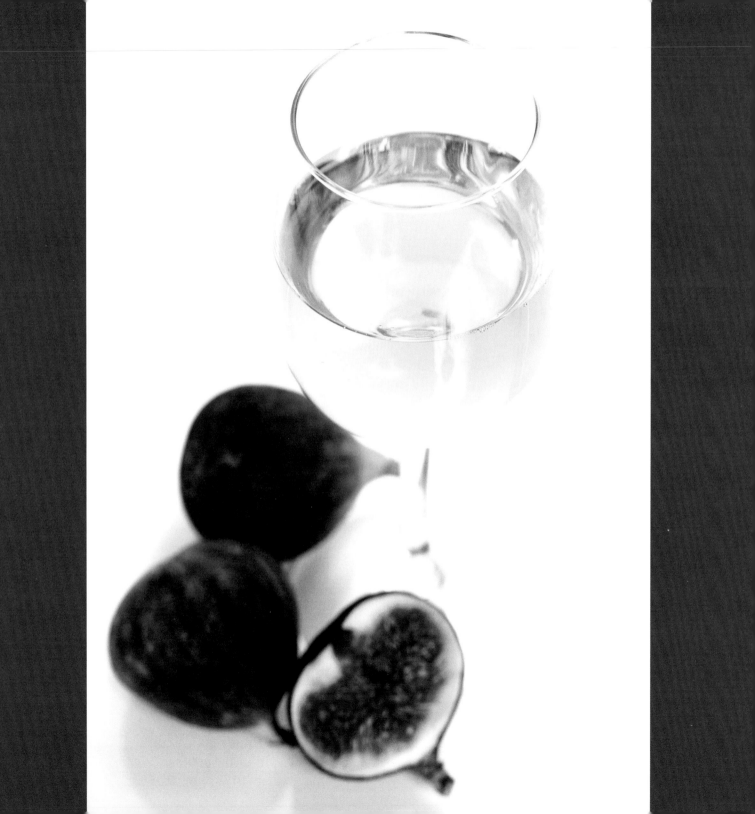

HALIBUT IN WINE & FIG MARINADE

*I*f you don't like fish, you can easily substitute the halibut for chicken breasts but be sure to fully cook your chicken, it generally takes much longer than fish.

- 6 skinless chunks of white halibut fish – approximately 6oz. each that are 1½ - 2" thick (so they don't fall apart)
- 5 garlic cloves – minced
- 1 tsp. salt
- 2 tsp. white pepper
- ¼ cup olive oil
- ¼ cup red wine vinegar

- ½ cup each of pitted prunes and dried figs, chopped into pieces
- ¼ cup of olives of choice (I like to use unpitted)
- ¼ cup Brown Sugar Splenda
- 1 cup of medium dry white wine
- 2 tbsp. fresh parsley – chopped

- ❖ Combine all ingredients except parsley and halibut in a bowl.
- ❖ Place halibut chunks in shallow baking dish. Pour mixture over halibut chunks and coat evenly.
- ❖ Cover baking dish and marinate halibut for 6 hours or overnight for best flavor. Flip halibut chunks a few times while marinating.
- ❖ Bake at 400° F for 35-45 minutes or until halibut is cooked thoroughly. Gently flip halibut once while cooking.
- ❖ Sprinkle with fresh parsley

I like to serve over brown basmati rice!

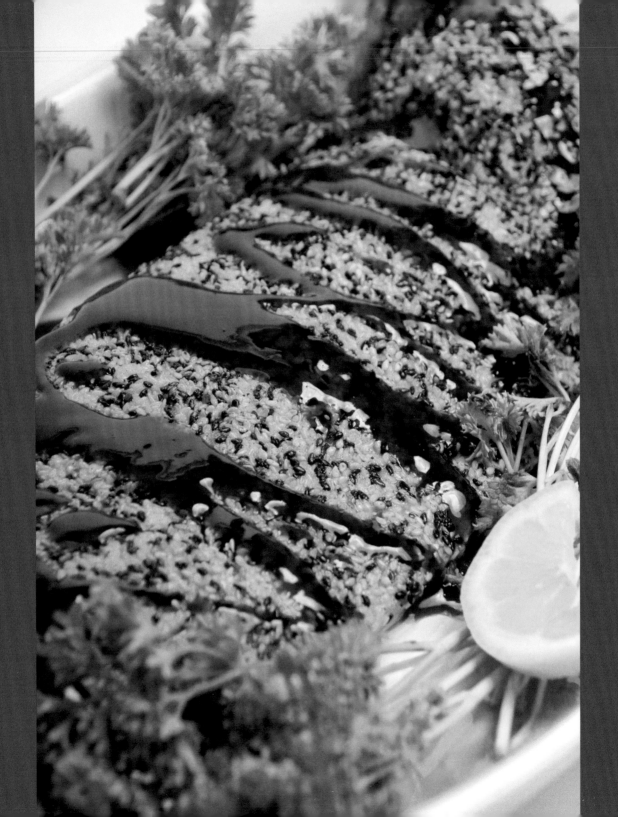

WASABI MAPLE SALMON

Salmon

- ▶ 5 tbsp. of toasted white and black sesame
- ▶ 1 large skinless salmon fillet or 5-6 chunks. You will need to use two flippers if you keep the fillet whole to prevent it from breaking apart. Even if it does break, you can arrange on dish and hide breaks with drizzled glaze.
- ▶ 2 tbsp. olive oil (this may be optional depending on type of salmon)
- ▶ course cracked pepper to taste

Wasabi Maple Glaze

- ▶ 3 tbsp. olive oil
- ▶ 4-5 tbsp. of wasabi paste (depending on how strong you like it)
- ▶ 1 tbsp. minced ginger
- ▶ 2 tbsp. of fresh lime juice
- ▶ 2 tbsp. of low sodium soy sauce
- ▶ ½ cup of 100% pure maple syrup

- ❖ Combine all sauce ingredients in a small saucepan and bring to a boil stirring constantly.
- ❖ Reduce heat and simmer on med-low heat until sauce reduces and thickens, whisking often.   If it gets too thick, you can add a little water to thin sauce.
- ❖ Keep sauce warm over low heat while preparing salmon… whisking occasionally
- ❖ Sauté salmon fillet(s) in olive oil on high heat using a large frying pan.
- ❖ Slightly brown both sides of salmon, reduce heat to medium low, add some cracked pepper and sesame seeds, cover and cook until salmon reaches desired doneness. I like salmon done medium-well so I cook salmon for approximately another 15 minutes after browning.
- ❖ Once salmon is done, place the whole fillet on a serving plate or dish out individual fillets of salmon and drizzle with the prepared wasabi glaze. Serve immediately.

I like this dish with sautéed veggies such as green beans, broccoli and cauliflower in a touch of sesame oil, lime juice, molasses and soy sauce.

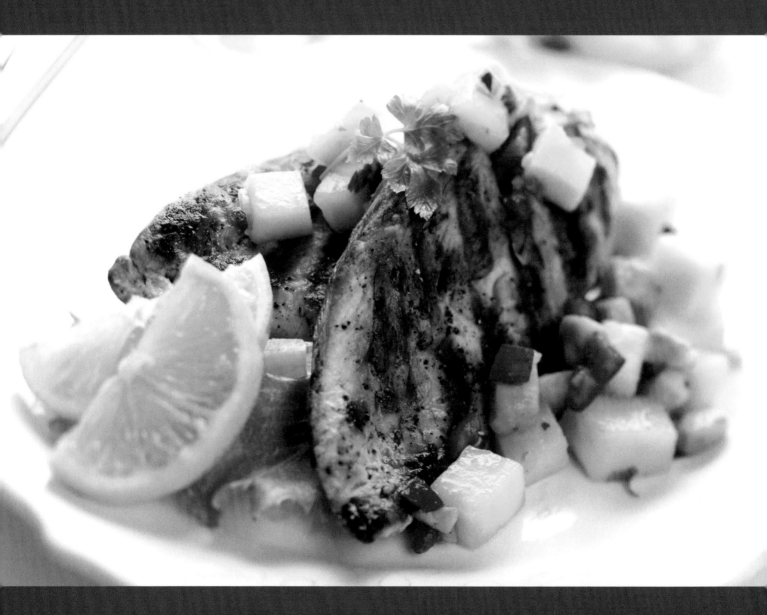

BBQ CHILI, LIME & BEER CHICKEN WITH MANGO SALSA

Chicken & Marinade

- ▶ 3lbs. of boneless/skinless chicken breasts
- ▶ 1 can of light beer
- ▶ Juice and pulp of one lime
- ▶ 3 cloves of garlic – minced

- ▶ 3 tbsp. of chili powder (I like to use organic Mexican chili powder)
- ▶ 1 tbsp. of salt
- ▶ 2 tsp. each of garlic powder, dehydrated onion
- ▶ 2 tbsp. of fancy molasses

Chicken Rub

- ▶ 4 tbsp. olive oil
- ▶ 4 tbsp. fresh lime juice
- ▶ 2 tbsp. fancy molasses

- ▶ 2 tsp. each of garlic powder, chili powder, ground dry mustard, salt, dried parsley, coriander, turmeric

- ❖ Combine all chicken marinade ingredients in a mixing bowl
- ❖ Using 2 extra-large Ziploc freezer bags, pour ½ of the marinade mixture in each bag.

- ❖ Place ½ of the chicken breasts in each bag of marinade

- ❖ Marinate for at least 6 hours or overnight.

- ❖ Combine Chicken Rub ingredients together in small bowl

- ❖ When chicken pieces are done marinating, remove chicken from Ziploc bags, pat dry and place on plate. Optional: pour marinade into small skillet for beer reduction (see directions below)

- ❖ Using a braising brush, brush some Chicken Rub over each piece of chicken.

- ❖ Place chicken on a BBQ or grill (can also be baked in the oven) and cook over medium heat.

- ❖ Optional: While chicken is cooking, heat marinade in skillet on stovetop until it comes to a boil. Reduce heat and simmer until liquid becomes thicker and is reduced to 1/3 of original volume.

- ❖ Cook chicken until meat thermometer registers well done for poultry. Remove chicken from BBQ or grill and if prepared - use 1-2 tbsp. of marinade reduction on each piece of chicken.

Serve with fresh mango salsa (recipe on next page) and sliced avocado for garnish. I like to have this dish with baked yam fries or a garden salad.

Remember....If you don't take time for your health, you'll eventually have to take time for illness

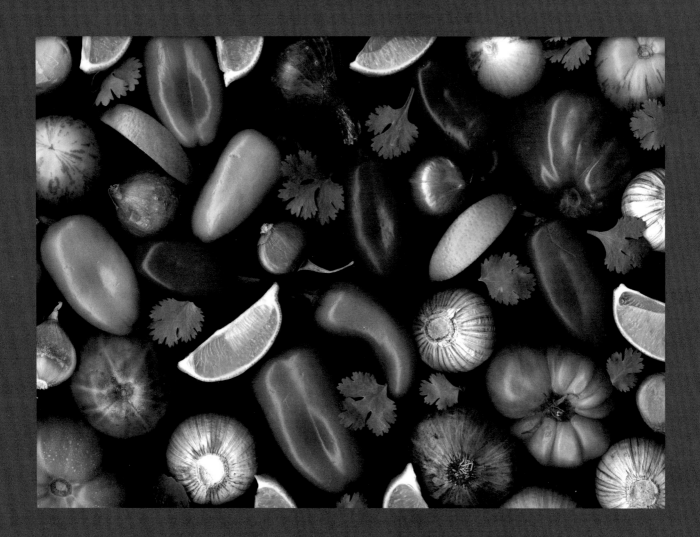

FRESH MANGO SALSA

*T*his recipe can be served with the BBQ Chili, Lime & Beer Chicken or any meal you like

- ► 2 fresh mangos – peeled and diced into small pieces

- ► 1 red pepper – diced

- ► 1 yellow pepper – diced

- ► 1 green pepper - diced

- ► 1 large red onion – diced

- ► ½ cup chopped green onion or chives

- ► 1 cup of cilantro – washed, dried and chopped

- ► 6 jalapeno slices or banana peppers from a jar with 1 tbsp. of the juice

- ► 1 tbsp. chili powder

- ► 1 ½ tsp. of salt

- ► 2 tbsp. of fresh squeezed lime juice

- ❖ Add all ingredients to a plastic or glass dish with a lid.

- ❖ Cover and shake to toss all ingredients together. Can be refrigerated for up to two days.

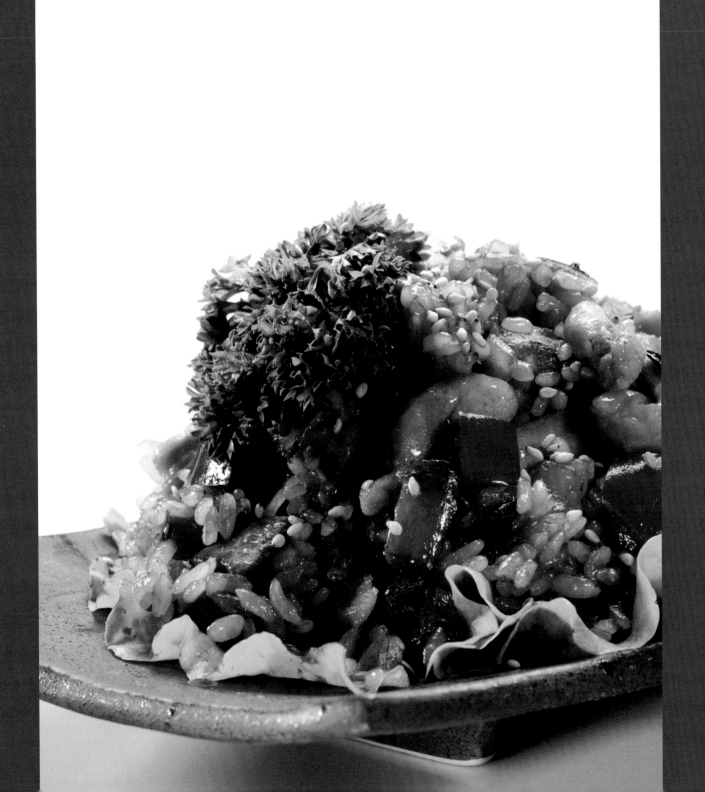

STIR FRY RICE

- 4 cups of cooked brown rice – at room temperature
- 4 boneless skinless chicken breasts – diced
- 3 tbsp. olive oil
- 1 large onion – diced
- 1 red pepper - diced
- 2 stalks of celery – diced
- 3 cloves of garlic – minced
- 1 cup of fresh mushrooms, sliced or diced
- 1 cup frozen peas
- 1 cup of shredded cabbage
- 1 cup of organic chicken broth – prepared
- 4 tbsp. of low sodium soy sauce
- 1 tbsp. of fancy molasses
- Pepper to taste
- Toasted sesame seeds and parsley to garnish
- 3 cups cooked rice of choice

- ❖ Sauté chicken pieces in olive oil over high heat for 5-7 minutes until slightly brown, add onion, red pepper, celery, garlic, mushrooms, peas, cabbage and ¼ cup of the chicken broth. Continue to sauté on medium-high to high heat until veggies are all tender and chicken is cooked thoroughly – approximately another 8-10 minutes. While mixture is cooking, prepare sauce in next step.

- ❖ Sauce: Combine the rest of the chicken broth, soy sauce, pepper and molasses in a bowl

- ❖ Lower heat to medium-low, stir in sauce and cooked rice until ingredients are combined and heated thoroughly.

- ❖ Garnish with fresh parsley if desired

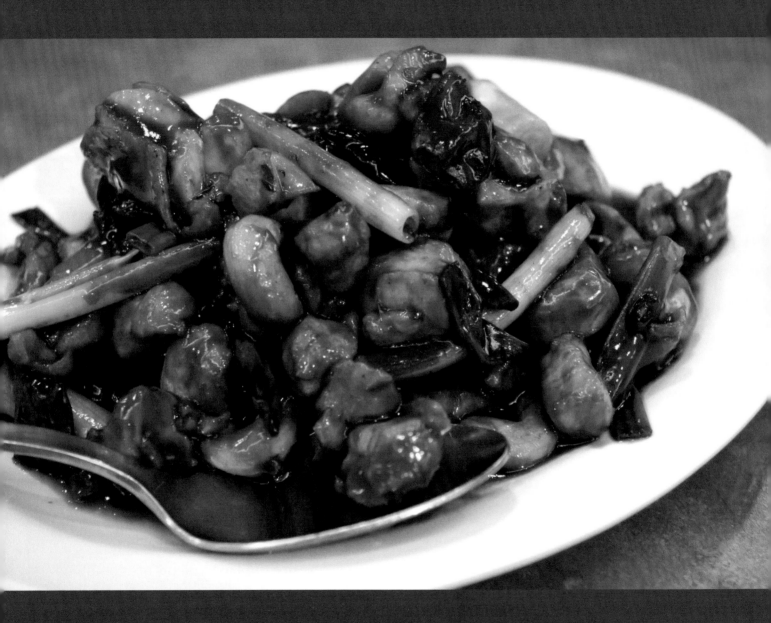

CHICKEN & CASHEWS WITH RICE NOODLES

- ► 1 pkg. of brown vermicelli rice noodles or 2 cups favorite rice

- ► 3 tbsp. sesame oil

- ► 2 lbs. of boneless skinless chicken breast – cut into bite size pieces

- ► 4 cups of diced veggies such as mushrooms, peppers, green onions or chives and cabbage

- ► ½ cup raw cashews

- ► ½ bunch of green onions or chives cut into thirds(long pieces)

Sauce

- ► 1 tbsp. Hoisin sauce (available in Asian food section of most grocery stores)

- ► ½ cup of organic chicken broth

- ► 1 cup unsweetened pineapple juice

- ► Juice and pulp from ½ fresh lime

- ► 3 tbsp. soy sauce

- ► 1 tbsp. of fancy molasses

- ► 2 tsp. chili paste (available in asian section of grocery store)

- ❖ Prepare vermicelli rice noodles or favorite rice as per package directions. The noodles are the very thin Asian style noodles usually found in the Asian section of most grocery stores – you can also use the white rice noodles if you can't find the brown rice ones.

- ❖ Prepare sauce by combining all ingredients together into a small saucepan. Heat sauce over medium heat and continue cooking until mixture reduces and becomes slightly thick. While sauce is cooking, go to next step.

❖ Sauté chicken in sesame oil over medium high heat so chicken becomes golden on the outside. Continue cooking over medium-low heat for approximately 10 minutes until chicken is almost thoroughly cooked. Add all veggies, raw cashews and prepared sauce, continue cooking over medium-low heat until all veggies are tender and chicken is fully cooked.

❖ Serve immediately. I like to have with the brown rice vermicelli noodles but you could also serve over your favorite rice if you prefer.

SHRIMP & SCALLOPS IN WINE REDUCTION

- ▶ 3 tbsp. olive or grape seed oil

- ▶ 1 large onion- thinly sliced

- ▶ 2 celery stalks – sliced

- ▶ 4 cloves of garlic - minced

- ▶ 1 ½ tbsp. organic chicken broth base

- ▶ 1 tsp. each of fresh lemon & lime juice

- ▶ ½ bottle medium white wine – approx. 375ml or 1 ⅔ cups (don't be scared to use a little wine here and there in cooking - unless you have special considerations or health problems – it's much lower in calories and fat than using cream or butter. I used wine in my cooking while preparing for a fitness competition and still ended up winning!)

- ▶ 2 lbs. large jumbo peeled and deveined shrimp

- ▶ 1 lb. jumbo scallops

- ▶ 2 cups cooked brown or white Asian style vermicelli rice noodles cooked per package directions. The noodles are found in Asian section of most grocery stores

- ▶ Salt, pepper and chili peppers to taste

- ▶ Fresh chopped parsley or cilantro to garnish

- ❖ Cook rice noodles as per package directions. If noodles aren't tender, boil noodles for 2-3 minutes until tender. Drain and set aside

- ❖ In medium frying pan, sauté onion, celery and garlic in olive oil over medium heat until veggies are tender

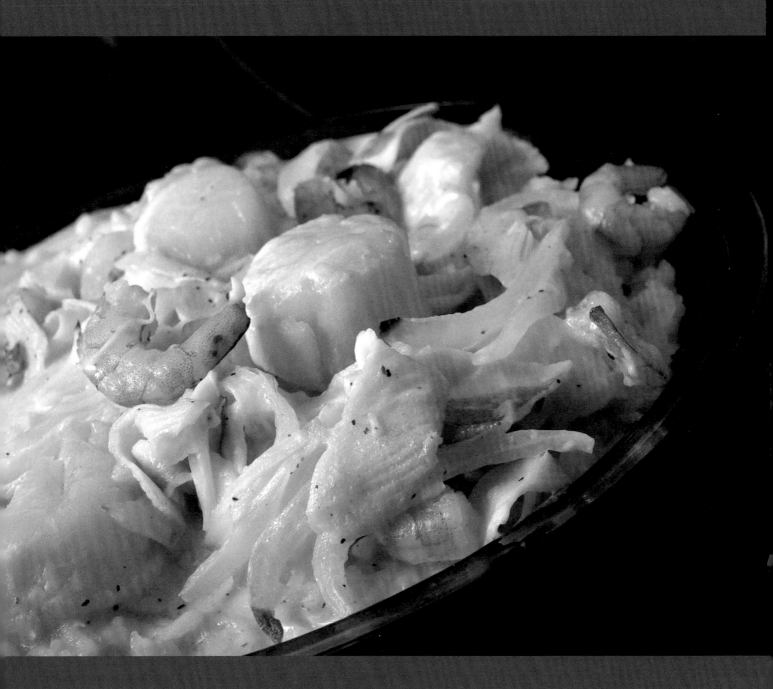

- ❖ Add the chicken base, lemon & lime juice and the wine

- ❖ Cook over medium-low heat (so wine is boiling slowly) until liquid is reduced to approx. ⅓ of original volume – this takes about 20 minutes

- ❖ Pat seafood dry, turn heat up to medium-high and add seafood to wine reduction. Cook until desired doneness, at least until shrimp are pink in color. I like to cook mine well – approx. 10 minutes.

- ❖ Add cooked and drained rice vermicelli noodles

- ❖ Season with salt, pepper and chili peppers, stir until combined

- ❖ Place on serving dish and garnish with parsley if you like

I like to have this dish with steamed veggies!

This recipe makes 4-6 servings depending on individual. If I was competing (as a 125 lb. female), I would have 1 cup of this yummy dish with 6-8 oz. of steamed veggies such as broccoli or cauliflower.

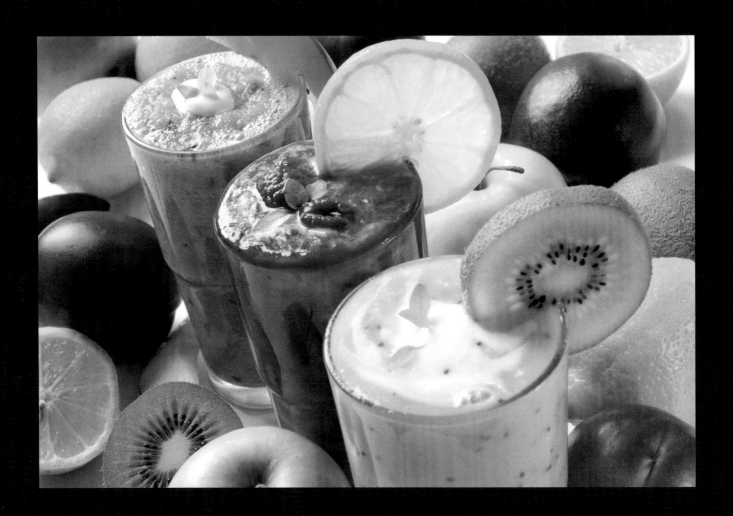

Smoothie Recipes

Can replace any meal of the day and great for when you are in a hurry

❖ Banana Nut Smoothie 93

❖ Orange & Pineapple Creamsicle 95

❖ Very Berry 97

❖ Chocolate Delight 98

❖ Coconut Cream Pie 99

❖ Monkey's Lunch 100

❖ Go Bananas 101

❖ Spinach Ginger & Kiwi 103

❖ Pumpkin Pie 104

SMOOTHIE RECIPE SECTION

I often use smoothies to replace a meal if I don't have time to cook and generally will have a smoothie for my post weight workout meal, it's a good way for me to ensure that I'm getting enough protein. You can make any of these for your children but would not recommend using protein powder for kids unless your health professional has recommended it.

There are a few tricks I use to make smoothies rich, thick, and delicious without all the extra calories.

Using frozen ingredients makes for a smoothie that tastes more like a milkshake. I always pre-slice and freeze ripe bananas in Ziploc bags so I have plenty on hand. I also like to pre-portion pure canned pumpkin in tiny containers that I can use in my pumpkin-pie smoothie. Frozen berries and spinach are great to use as well. You can hardly taste the spinach when it's mixed with other things.

You can use a small blender or blender bullet– I really like the Hamilton Beach Single Shot Blender, it works quite well!

To keep smoothies lower in calories I use the Unsweetened Almond Breeze or Coconut/Almond Dream which comes in a one liter carton. These are 40-60 calories per cup so no need to worry about extra calories. I sometimes use ½ unsweetened juice and ½ of the Almond Breeze or Coconut Dream. For my kids, I use regular low fat milk.

For protein powder, I generally use an all Natural 100% Whey Powder such as the IsoNatural. I find smoothies turn out better if you blend all the ingredients except the protein powder first and then add the protein at the end. If for any reason you don't like to use protein powder – you can substitute it for ½ cup of dry cottage cheese… Yes, cottage cheese blends up quite well and offers a great protein source!

BANANA NUT SMOOTHIE

- ▶ 1 small frozen banana – I usually peel and slice my ripe bananas and then freeze in Ziploc bags - I like this much better than using fresh

- ▶ 3-4 ice cubes

- ▶ 1 tbsp. all natural peanut, cashew or almond butter

- ▶ 1 tsp. vanilla extract

- ▶ Unsweetened Almond Breeze or Coconut Dream (60 calories per cup) to cover ice – Or you can use skim milk if preferred

- ▶ 1 scoop of all natural vanilla, plain or banana flavored protein powder

- ▶ Splenda or other no-calorie sweetener to taste (optional)

- ❖ Place all ingredients except protein powder in a small blender.

- ❖ Blend until all ingredients are blended together.

- ❖ Add protein powder and blend another 30-40 seconds.

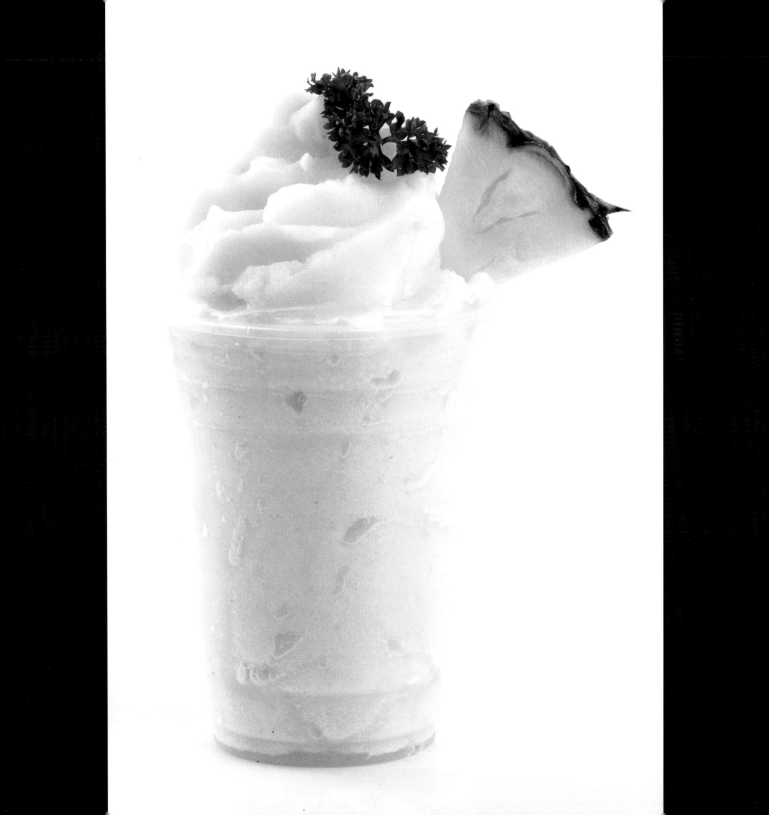

ORANGE & PINEAPPLE CREAMSICLE

- ► 2 tbsp. unsweetened concentrated frozen orange juice

- ► 6 bite size chunks of pineapple (frozen is best)

- ► 3-4 ice cubes

- ► 1 tsp. all natural vanilla extract

- ► ½ tsp. orange extract

- ► Unsweetened almond milk or Coconut Dream (60 calories per cup) to cover ice – Or you can use skim milk if preferred

- ► 1 scoop of all natural vanilla, plain or orange flavored protein powder

- ► Splenda or other no-calorie sweetener to taste (optional)

- ❖ Place all ingredients except protein powder in a small blender.

- ❖ Blend until all ingredients are blended together.

- ❖ Add protein powder and blend another 30-40 seconds.

Garnish with fresh sliced pineapple and oranges if you wish… a summer delight!!

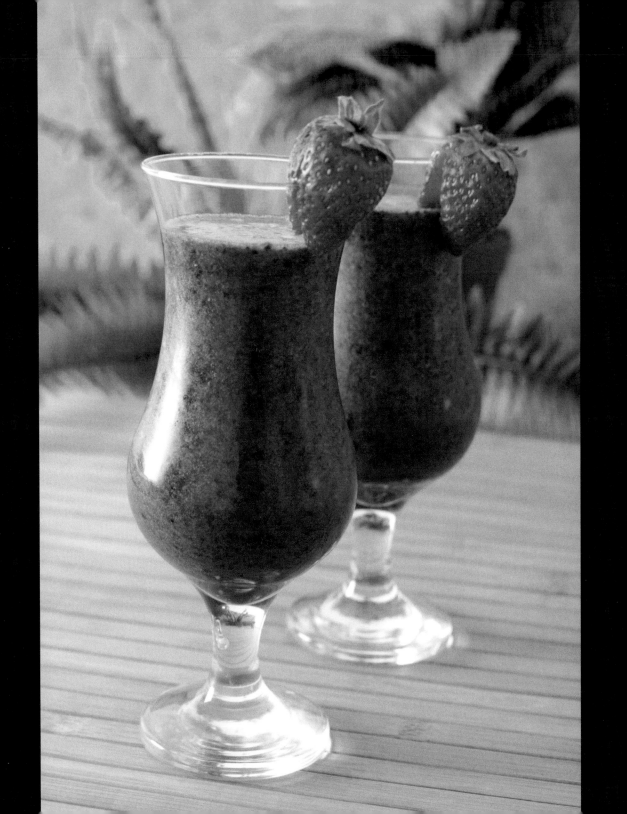

VERY BERRY

- ► ¾ cup frozen mixed berries

- ► ½ cup unsweetened fruit juice – I like to use a blend

- ► Unsweetened almond milk or Coconut Dream (60 calories per cup) to cover ingredients – or you can use skim milk if preferred

- ► 1 scoop of all natural vanilla, plain or berry flavored protein powder

- ► Splenda or other no-calorie sweetener to taste (optional)

- ❖ Place all ingredients except protein powder in a small blender.

- ❖ Blend until all ingredients are blended together.

- ❖ Add protein powder and blend another 30-40 seconds.

CHOCOLATE DELIGHT

- ▶ 5-6 ice cubes

- ▶ 2 tbsp. cocoa powder

- ▶ ½ cup sugar free chocolate pudding or sugar free ice cream (optional)

- ▶ Unsweetened almond milk or Coconut Dream (60 calories per cup) to cover ice – Or you can use skim milk if preferred

- ▶ 1 scoop of all natural vanilla, plain or chocolate flavored protein powder

- ▶ Splenda or other no-calorie sweetener to taste (optional)

- ❖ Place all ingredients except protein powder in a small blender.

- ❖ Blend until all ingredients are blended together.

- ❖ Add protein powder and blend another 30-40 seconds.

COCONUT CREAM PIE

- ▶ 4-5 ice cubes

- ▶ ½ cup coconut flavored dessert tofu (if you can't find this you can blend together ½ cup no fat Greek yogurt with 2 tbsp. unsweetened shredded coconut)

- ▶ 1 tsp of coconut flavored extract

- ▶ ½ cup pure coconut water

- ▶ Coconut Dream(low fat coconut milk – 60cal per cup) to cover ingredients

- ▶ 1 scoop of all natural vanilla or plain protein powder

- ▶ Splenda or other no-calorie sweetener to taste (optional)

- ❖ Place all ingredients except protein powder in a small blender.

- ❖ Blend until all ingredients are blended together.

- ❖ Add protein powder and blend another 30-40 seconds.

MONKEY'S LUNCH

- ▶ 1 small sliced frozen banana
- ▶ 2-3 ice cubes
- ▶ 2 tbsp. chocolate cocoa powder
- ▶ 1 tbsp. all natural peanut butter
- ▶ Unsweetened almond milk or Coconut Dream (60 calories per cup) to cover ice – or you can use skim milk if preferred
- ▶ 1 scoop of all natural vanilla, plain or chocolate flavored protein powder
- ▶ Splenda or other no-calorie sweetener to taste (optional)

❖ Place all ingredients except protein powder in a small blender.

❖ Blend until all ingredients are blended together.

❖ Add protein powder and blend another 30-40 seconds.

GO BANANAS

- ▶ 1 small sliced frozen banana

- ▶ ½ cup no fat banana flavored pudding, yogurt or tofu

- ▶ 1 tsp. banana extract

- ▶ Unsweetened almond milk or Coconut Dream (60 calories per cup)

- to cover ice – or you can use skim milk if preferred

- ▶ 1 scoop of all natural vanilla, plain or banana flavored protein powder

- ▶ Splenda or other no-calorie sweetener to taste (optional)

- ❖ Place all ingredients except protein powder in a small blender.

- ❖ Blend until all ingredients are blended together.

- ❖ Add protein powder and blend another 30-40 seconds.

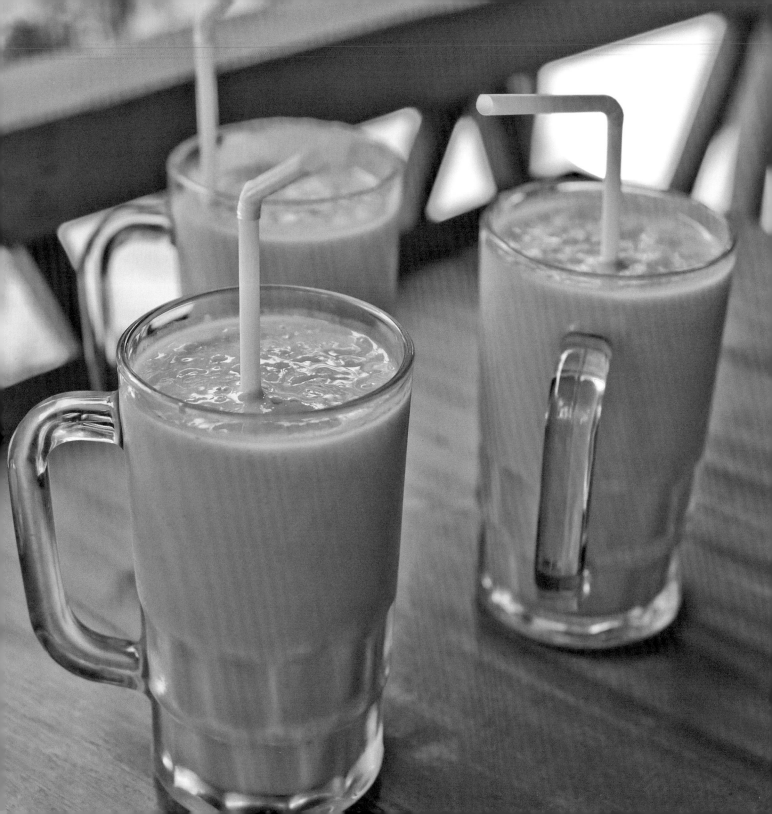

SPINACH GINGER & KIWI

This may not sound so appealing but it really is quite yummy and full of nutritious stuff!!

- ▶ 1 cup frozen spinach leaves – I usually buy a big container and portion one cup into zip loc bags to freeze.

- ▶ 1 small apple, cored with seeds out

- ▶ 1 small kiwi, can use frozen if you have some and can also keep the peel on if you like

- ▶ 1 tbsp. minced ginger, can keep the peel on if you like

- ▶ ½ cup unsweetened apple juice

- ▶ ½ small sliced frozen banana

- ▶ Unsweetened almond milk or Coconut Dream (60 calories per cup) to cover ice – Or you can use skim milk if preferred

- ▶ 1 scoop of all natural vanilla or plain protein powder

- ▶ Splenda or other no-calorie sweetener to taste (optional)

- ❖ Place all ingredients except protein powder in a small blender.

- ❖ Blend until all ingredients are blended together.

- ❖ Add protein powder and blend another 30-40 seconds.

PUMPKIN PIE

- ▶ 1/3 cup pure canned pumpkin – frozen in little container. I usually microwave for 30 seconds so pumpkin will come out of container into blender.

- ▶ 2-3 ice cubes

- ▶ 2 tbsp. of pumpkin spice

- ▶ 1 tsp. vanilla extract

- ▶ Unsweetened almond milk or Coconut Dream (60 calories per cup) to cover ice – Or you can use skim milk if preferred

- ▶ 1 scoop of all natural vanilla or flavored protein powder

- ▶ Splenda or other no-calorie sweetener to taste (optional)

❖ Place all ingredients except protein powder in a small blender.

❖ Blend until all ingredients are blended together.

❖ Add protein powder and blend another 30-40 seconds.

Remember...Live, Love, Laugh & Eat Well

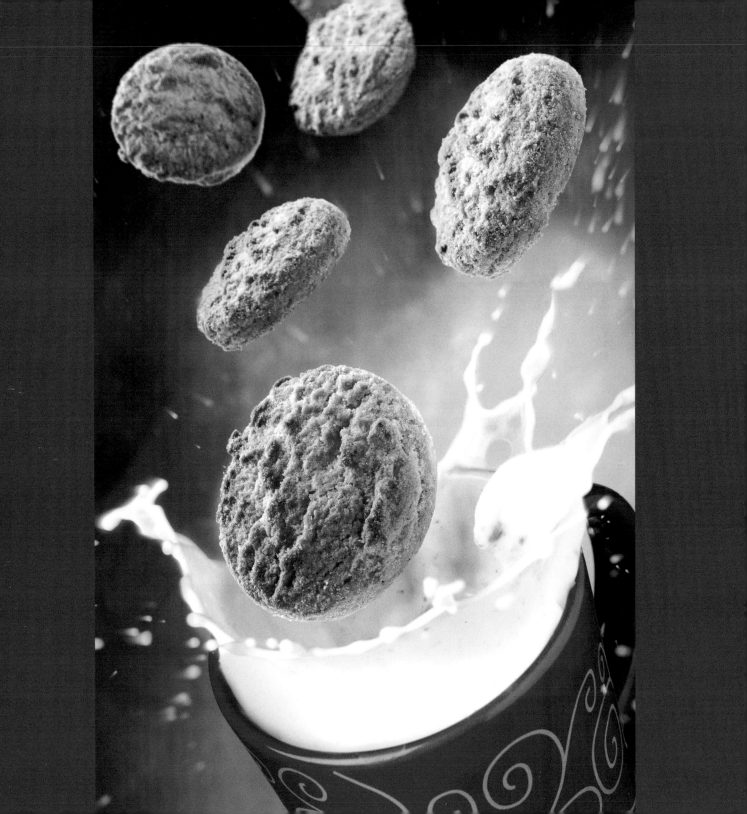

Tasty Treat Section

Can use to replace any meal of the day... Very convenient if you're on the go.

❖ Pumpkin Ginger Cookies 109

❖ Oatmeal Raisin Protein Cookies 111

❖ Peanut Butter & Oat Cookies 112

❖ Banana Protein Loaf 113

❖ Apple Zucchini Muffins 114

❖ Protein, Carrot & Flax Muffins 117

❖ Pecan & Apricot Energy Bars 118

❖ Peanut Butter Balls 119

TASTY TREATS

*T*f you have a sweet tooth like I do… you are going to love having some of these stocked up in your freezer, ready to eat! I quite often use these for my first meal with my coffee in the morning or between lunch and dinner.

Although I refer to the recipes in this section as Tasty Treats…. You could use them to replace any meal of the day as the recipes in this section contain the major food groups including healthy carbohydrates and protein. Many of the recipes have some fruit or veggies in them as well! These recipes are great for people with hectic work schedules or who travel a lot… especially if you crave cookies and treats. The difference is that most of these treats have no added sugar and include lots of healthy ingredients!

PUMPKIN GINGER COOKIES

- 3 ½ cups of old fashioned oats
- 1 ½ cups of all natural plain whey powder
- 2 ½ cups of Splenda or other 0 calorie sweetener
- ½ cup coconut oil (great for baking) or olive oil
- ½ tsp. salt
- 2 tbsp. of grated or minced ginger (optional)

- 1 ½ tbsp. pumpkin spice
- 1 ¼ cups pure pumpkin puree
- 1 ½ cups unsweetened applesauce
- 1 ½ cups unsweetened raisins
- 1/3 cup liquid egg whites
- 1 tbsp. vanilla extract
- 2 tbsp. fancy molasses (optional)

❖ Preheat oven to 350° F

❖ Lightly spray cooking sheet with cooking spray

❖ Crumble first seven ingredients together until combined

❖ Mix rest of ingredients into crumbled ingredients until blended

❖ Drop by tablespoons onto baking sheet (the type of baking sheet and cooking spray can greatly affect texture of cookie – I use the Western Family Cooking Spray)

❖ Bake for 13-15 minutes

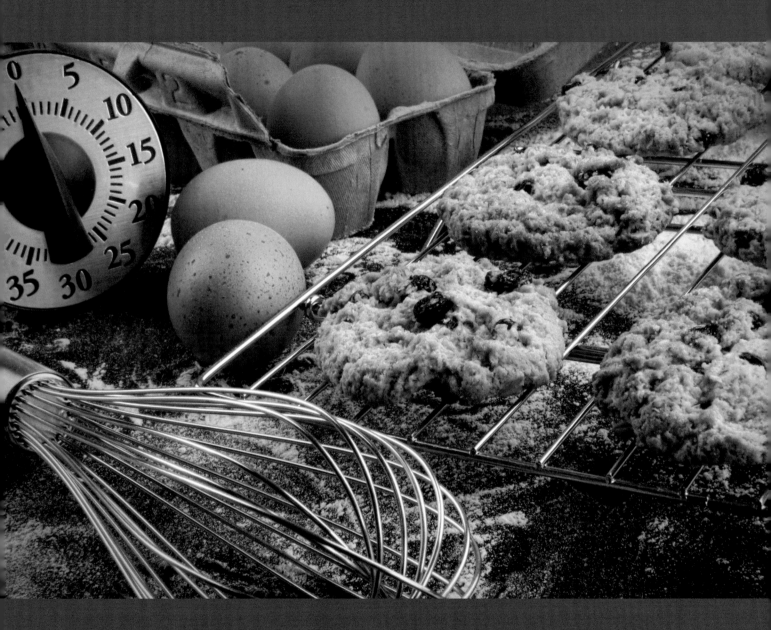

OATMEAL RAISIN PROTEIN COOKIES

- ▶ 3 tbsp. of coconut oil (great for baking) or olive oil

- ▶ 4 cups old fashioned oats

- ▶ 1 cup of all natural plain whey powder – the kind of whey powder you use will greatly affect the texture of these cookies

- ▶ 1 ½ cups of Splenda or other 0 calorie sweetener

- ▶ ¼ tsp. salt (optional)

- ▶ Cinnamon to taste

- ▶ 1 cup unsweetened raisins

- ▶ 1 cup liquid egg whites (the pure ones)

- ▶ 1 cup unsweetened applesauce

- ❖ Preheat oven to 325° F

- ❖ Spray cookie sheet with no fat cooking spray – the type of cookie sheet used will greatly affect the texture and baking time of these cookies, use a thick good quality cookie sheet.

- ❖ Crumble first six ingredients together with your hands until combined

- ❖ Add remaining ingredients and blend well

- ❖ Drop dough on to cookie sheet using large tablespoon

- ❖ Bake for 8-10 minutes – do not over bake or they will be dry

- ❖ Refrigerate cookies that you do not eat in the same day. They also freeze well

PEANUT BUTTER & OAT COOKIES

- ▶ 2 cups all natural peanut or almond butter
- ▶ ½ cup olive oil
- ▶ ½ tsp. salt
- ▶ 2 tbsp. baking soda
- ▶ 3 ½ cups old fashioned oats

- ▶ 1 cup of all natural plain whey powder
- ▶ 2 cups of Splenda or other 0 calorie sweetener
- ▶ ½ cup Brown Sugar Splenda
- ▶ ¾ cup liquid egg whites (the pure ones)
- ▶ 2 tbsp. fancy molasses

- ❖ Preheat oven to 350° F
- ❖ Lightly spray cooking sheet with cooking spray – use a good quality heavy duty cookie sheet for best results
- ❖ Combine first 4 ingredients together until smooth
- ❖ Add remainder ingredients and blend well
- ❖ Drop by tablespoons onto baking sheet
- ❖ Bake for 8-10 minutes

My kids absolutely love these although I make them with a real sugar such as brown or coconut sugar as I don't like to give them sugar substitutes.

BANANA PROTEIN LOAF

- ▶ 4 large ripe bananas – mashed
- ▶ 3/4 cup brown rice flour
- ▶ ½ cup old fashioned oats
- ▶ ½ cup plain protein powder
- ▶ 1/3 cup olive or melted coconut oil
- ▶ 1 cup Splenda or other 0 calorie sweetener
- ▶ 1 egg or 2 egg whites
- ▶ 1 tsp. vanilla extract
- ▶ 1 tsp. baking soda
- ▶ ¼ tsp. salt

- ❖ Preheat oven to 350° F
- ❖ Lightly grease loaf pan with no-fat cooking spray
- ❖ Mash bananas in large bowl
- ❖ Add remaining ingredients and mix with fork until well combined
- ❖ Pour into loaf pan
- ❖ Bake for 35-40 minutes or until toothpick inserted in middle of loaf comes out clean
- ❖ Cool slightly and then tip upside down on cooling rack
- ❖ Wait until loaf is completely cooled to slice

When I'm not competing, I like to add a few carob or dark chocolate chips to this recipe!

APPLE ZUCCHINI MUFFINS

- ► 1 cup oat flour
- ► ½ cup brown rice flour
- ► ½ cup all natural plain whey powder
- ► 1 ½ tsp. baking powder
- ► 1 ½ tsp. baking soda
- ► ½ tsp. cinnamon
- ► ¼ tsp. salt
- ► 1 cup Splenda
- ► 2 tbsp. of coconut oil or oil of choice
- ► 5 egg whites

- ► ¾ cup plain yogurt (can use no-fat if you wish)
- ► ¾ cup unsweetened applesauce
- ► 1 tsp. lemon juice
- ► 1 tsp. vanilla extract
- ► 1 ½ cups grated zucchini with peel on
- ► 2 cups grated apples with or without peel

- ❖ Preheat oven to 350° F
- ❖ Lightly spray non- stick muffin tins – I spray the top of pan as well
- ❖ Mix all dry ingredients together
- ❖ Add oil and crumble together with hands

- ❖ Add remaining ingredients except zucchini and apples and mix well
- ❖ Fold in zucchini and apples just until blended
- ❖ Bake 20 minutes or until muffins are cooked in middle
- ❖ Carefully loosen edges of muffins from tin
- ❖ Place upside down on cooling rack to cool
- ❖ Remove muffins and enjoy!!

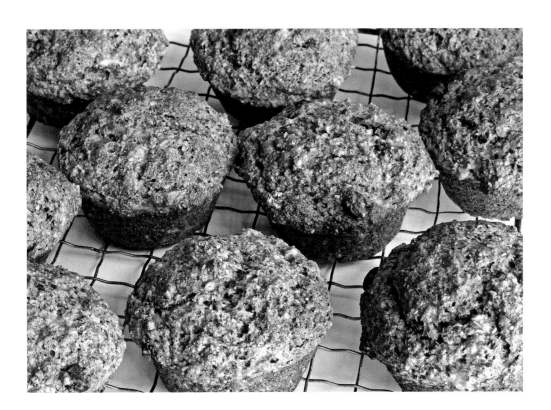

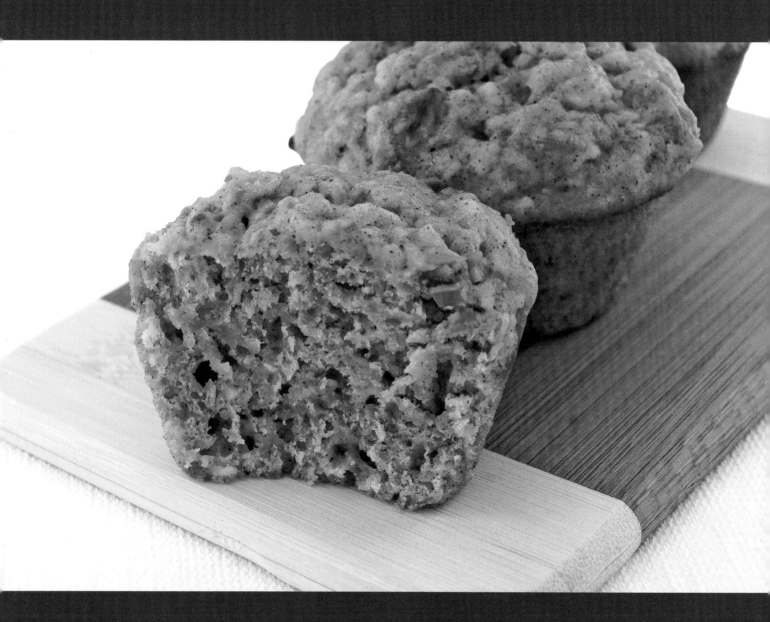

PROTEIN, CARROT & FLAX MUFFINS

- ▶ 1 cup oat flour
- ▶ 1 cup all natural plain whey powder
- ▶ 8 tbsp. flax or chia seeds
- ▶ 1 tsp. baking powder
- ▶ 1 tsp. baking soda
- ▶ 1 tsp. each of cinnamon, nutmeg and pumpkin spice

- ▶ ½ tsp. salt
- ▶ 2 cups egg whites
- ▶ 1 cup pure canned pumpkin
- ▶ 1 cup Splenda or other 0 calorie sweetener
- ▶ ¾ cup unsweetened applesauce
- ▶ ½ cup grated carrots

- ❖ Preheat oven to 350° F
- ❖ Lightly spray non-stick muffin tins with cooking spray
- ❖ Mix all dry ingredients together
- ❖ Add remaining ingredients and stir until blended
- ❖ Pour into muffin tins
- ❖ Bake 12-15 minutes until baked thoroughly
- ❖ Carefully loosen edges of muffins from tin
- ❖ Place upside down on cooling rack to cool
- ❖ Remove muffins and enjoy!!

PECAN & APRICOT ENERGY BARS

- ▶ 2 cups all natural peanut, almond or cashew butter
- ▶ ¾ cup honey
- ▶ ¼ cup fancy molasses
- ▶ ½ cup unsweetened applesauce
- ▶ ½ cup Splenda or other 0 calorie sweetener
- ▶ ½ cup kamut flakes

- ▶ ½ cup all natural plain whey powder
- ▶ 1 cup old fashioned oats
- ▶ 1 cup brown crisped rice cereal (found in health food stores)
- ▶ 1 cup chopped raw pecans
- ▶ 1 cup chopped unsweetened dried apricots

- ❖ Line square glass pan with parchment paper, leave excess paper hanging on sides of pan so you can pull out the whole pan of energy bars in one piece.

- ❖ Melt nut butter slightly in a large dish so it mixes easily, you can do this in microwave

- ❖ Add remaining ingredients to nut butter and mix well

- ❖ Press into lined square pan

- ❖ Use parchment paper on top to press ingredients into pan

- ❖ Place pan in freezer for two hours

- ❖ Remove from pan using sides of parchment paper, place onto cutting board and cut into small squares. Place into airtight freezer container and freeze

- ❖ Keep frozen until ready to eat. These can be eaten directly from freezer or thaw for a few minutes if you prefer

PEANUT BUTTER BALLS

- ▶ 2 ½ cups all natural peanut butter mixed with 1/3 cup of vegan or olive oil margarine – whip together until combined

- ▶ 1 cup chocolate peanut butter or vanilla protein powder

- ▶ ½ cup Splenda or other no calorie sweetener

- ▶ ¼ cup Brown Sugar Splenda substitute

- ▶ 1 ½ cups brown crisped rice cereal (found in health stores)

- ❖ Ensure peanut butter and margarine are whipped together with electric mixer until well blended

- ❖ Add remaining ingredients together and blend well

- ❖ Form into small balls by squeezing approx. 2 tbsp. of the mixture in your hand until it is formed and then roll gently between palms to round into ball shape

- ❖ Place on parchment paper and put into freezer for two hours

- ❖ Eat immediately or freeze in airtight freezer container until ready to eat

My husband's fav!! We eat them right out of the freezer!

MY FITNESS CAREER

2013	Wrote my first fitness recipe book - thank-you for purchasing!!
2013	Selected for Shapefit's Model of the Week
2013	Became Certified As A Specialist In Fitness Nutrition
2011	Appeared in Oxygen magazine (Fit Moms Section)
2010	Opened a Lakefront Fitness Studio
2009	Appeared in Oxygen magazine (Future of Fitness)
2009	Obtained Pro Status as a Fitness Model
2009	1st place Advanced Fitness Model, FAME West, Vancouver BC
2009	Obtained my Personal Trainer Certification, ISSA
2009	5th place, Figure, WBFF BC Championships
2008	On-line articles published for Urban Male Magazine
2008	7th place, Advanced Fitness Model, FAME Worlds (Toronto, ON)
2008	1st place, Open Fitness Model, FAME Regional (Calgary, AB)
1996	Became a Certified Dietary Technologist